D1121764

THE INSULIN RESISTANCE SOLUTION

Reverse Pre-Diabetes

Repair Your Metabolism | Shed Belly Fat | Prevent Diabetes

ROB THOMPSON, M.D.
author of *The Glycemic-Load Diet*

with more than 75 recipes by
DANA CARPENDER

FAIR WINDS

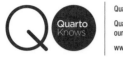

Quarto is the authority on a wide range of topics.

Quarto educates, entertains and enriches the lives of our readers—enthusiasts and lovers of hands-on living.

www.QuartoKnows.com

First published in the United States of America in 2016 by
Fair Winds Press, an imprint of
Quarto Publishing Group USA Inc.
100 Cummings Center
Suite 406-L
Beverly, Massachusetts 01915-6101
Telephone: (978) 282-9590
Fax: (978) 283-2742
QuartoKnows.com
Visit our blogs at QuartoKnows.com

20 19 18 17 16   1 2 3 4 5

ISBN: 978-1-59233-646-3
Digital edition published in 2016
eISBN: 978-1-62788-190-6

Library of Congress Cataloging-in-Publication Data available.

Interior page design: *tabula rasa* graphic design
Printed in the USA

The information in this book is for educational purposes only. It is not intended to replace the advice of a physician or medical practitioner. Please see your health care provider before beginning any new health program.

To my patients, who have always placed their trust in me.
Rob Thompson, M.D.

This one I dedicate to you, readers. You have
been given bad advice, and it has led you to a
dangerous place. That changes today. Welcome to
the rest of your life—you are going to be amazed.
Dana Carpender

CONTENTS

Part III

Recipes and Meal Plans
for Reducing Insulin Resistance by Dana Carpender   **82**

INTRODUCTION

BELLY FAT—
THE CANARY IN THE COAL MINE

You don't like the way you look. Your clothes don't fit, you can't move around as easily as you used to. Maybe your doctor said you're at risk for diabetes. But what can you do? You've tried diets. They work for a while, and then the weight comes creeping back. You blame it on a lack of self-discipline, but consider this: twice as many Americans are overweight now than forty years ago. Did all these people suddenly just lose their willpower? It doesn't make sense. Why should you deprive yourself, when people forty years ago seemed to be able to eat what they wanted without getting fat?

Back then, Americans figured they were on track to be healthier than ever, but then something happened that ended up making us less healthy. Scientists thought they had discovered what caused heart attacks: the cholesterol in food. They also thought they knew what caused obesity: eating too much fat. They spread the word that if you wanted to stay slim and prevent heart disease, you needed to avoid foods containing fat and cholesterol, including eggs, dairy products, red meat, and fatty vegetables such as nuts, olives, and avocados. Grocery stores responded by selling low-fat, low-cholesterol foods; vegetarianism became popular; and for the first time in history, the U.S. Food and Drug Administration (FDA) got involved in trying to get people to "eat right"—i.e., consume less fat and cholesterol. Americans did what they were told: from 1970 to 1997, they reduced their consumption of eggs by 23 percent; milk fat by 52 percent; and red meat by 16 percent.

Well, we *are* living longer, but it's not because we changed our diet. Fewer of us are smoking, and we have better treatments for heart disease, cancer, and stroke. But the fact is, we're still an unhealthy lot. Two-thirds of us are overweight, a third are obese, and, since 1970, the diabetes rate has *tripled*. More of us than ever suffer from arthritis and gout. More men complain of reduced vitality and sex drive, and more women are battling infertility. Despite all the advances in medicine that have been made in the last fifty years, we don't look as good as we should, we don't feel as good as we should, and we're suffering from serious medical problems at higher rates than ever.

We're also shaped differently than we were before; our bellies are bigger. Obviously, if you gain weight your belly will get bigger, but studies show that the sizes of our abdomens relative to the rest of our bodies are increasing. Even skinny folks these days have potbellies. Since 2002, our average weight has stayed the same, but our bellies have gotten even bigger.

What's causing these problems? The tip-off is the potbelly. Belly fat is the proverbial canary in the coal mine, a sign that something is making us sick. Only it's not coal mine gas causing the trouble. It's one of our own hormones—*insulin.* We're producing too much of it, and it's bringing on a host of problems that were much less common forty years ago, including abdominal obesity, adult-onset diabetes, female infertility, and low testosterone in men.

The problem is what doctors call *insulin resistance.* It sounds technical, but it's pretty simple. Your body needs insulin to transport the glucose out of your bloodstream into your muscles. If you have insulin resistance, your muscles lose their responsiveness to insulin—they become resistant to insulin. As a result, your insulin-making cells—the *beta cells* of your pancreas—have to produce larger than normal amounts of insulin to control your blood glucose levels.

If you haven't heard of insulin resistance, that's understandable. It has only been in the past decade or so that doctors have learned how to diagnosis it and discovered how common it is. America is experiencing an epidemic of insulin resistance. Approximately a third of the American population develops it by the time they turn forty. This epidemic has turned previous thinking about diet on its head. No longer does the FDA recommend reducing dietary fat and cholesterol. The emphasis of the latest Dietary Guidelines for Americans is on reversing insulin resistance.

The good news is that insulin resistance is actually easy to prevent, treat, and reverse. In fact, in the past people avoided it without even trying. You don't need to go on a diet. You don't need to sweat and strain at a gym. You don't need to take medication. You just need to reduce the amount of insulin your body produces, and if you understand what's going on, this is remarkably easy to do.

Part I of this book will help you determine whether you have insulin resistance and explain how a few seemingly minor lifestyle changes can have major effects on how much insulin your body produces. Part II will show you how easy it is to regain your sensitivity to insulin and restore a normal hormone balance without dieting, in the usual sense of the word, or engaging in grueling exercise. Part III will deliver delicious recipes to put you on the path toward a healthier and tastier way of eating.

PART I

UNDERSTANDING INSULIN RESISTANCE

1

INSULIN: TOO MUCH OF A GOOD THING

Your body gets its fuel from three kinds of food: carbohydrates, protein, and fat. Carbohydrates are plant products such as fruits, vegetables, grains, and sugar. Fat and protein come from animal products, including eggs, meat, and dairy, and from fatty vegetables such as nuts, olives, and avocados. Each kind of food has its own building block. For carbohydrates, it's a type of sugar called *glucose*; for protein, *amino acids*; for fat, *fatty acids*. Your digestive system breaks down each kind of food to its basic building block before absorbing it into your bloodstream.

When these fuels enter the bloodstream, your body needs insulin to process the glucose from carbohydrates, but hardly any at all to handle the amino acids and fatty acids from animal products and fatty vegetables. The bottom line: the amount of insulin your body produces mainly depends on how many carbohydrates you eat.

CONFUSION ABOUT THE WORD SUGAR

Sugars—glucose, fructose, and sucrose—are natural parts of the human diet. Fruits and vegetables are full of them. They all taste sweet, and humans enjoy the taste of sweetness, which is why we like to add them to food. Unfortunately, doctors use the word *sugar* loosely, which causes a lot of confusion. When they talk about *blood sugar*, they mean glucose; the proper term is "blood glucose." When they talk about the sugar we add to sweeten food, such as the sugar in your sugar bowl, they mean sucrose. Sucrose is not the same as glucose. It's actually a double molecule of glucose and fructose. It's important to understand that most of the "sugar" in your blood (glucose) does not come from the "sugar" added to food (sucrose). It comes from the breakdown of carbohydrates—mainly refined carbohydrates such as bread, potatoes, rice, and pasta. When you read or hear that Americans are consuming too much sugar, often the media doesn't make it clear that this isn't from added sugar. It's mostly due to a rise in consumption of refined carbohydrates. Added sugar is a minor contributor and mainly a problem for children and teenagers who consume a lot of soda.

A RADICAL CHANGE IN THE HUMAN DIET

For millions of years, prehistoric humans lived mainly on fat and protein from eating other animals: large ones, small ones, fish, even bugs. The carbohydrates they ate—roots, bark, grasses, and the occasional piece of fruit—were full of vitamins, minerals, and fiber, but provided little in the way of calories. Now, we get more calories from carbohydrates—mainly grain products such as wheat and rice—than from any other kind of food. These carbohydrates were not part of the prehistoric diet. It's only in the past 10,000 years, a brief interval in the timeline of human existence, that humans have developed the means to extract the edible cores of grains from their husks and turn them into food.

Grains are full of *starch,* a concentrated form of glucose. Each molecule of starch contains hundreds of glucose molecules. As soon as starch reaches your intestines, your digestive enzymes unhitch those molecules and release pure glucose. The glucose in flour products, potatoes, rice, and corn now provide more calories to humans than any other kind of food.

Another source of glucose is sucrose, our favorite sweetener. Humans have always been attracted to sweetness. We have taste buds on our tongues that respond only to sugar. These served a purpose to prehistoric humans. A hint of sweetness in a bite of a plant meant it could provide calories and was safe to eat. Eventually, our ancestors learned how to extract pure sucrose from sugar cane. This was a rare delicacy until the nineteenth century, when sugar plantations began producing large quantities and it became a significant part of our diet. In the 1970s, food manufacturers developed more efficient ways of producing sugar by extracting it from corn—so-called high-fructose corn syrup. This made sugar-sweetened beverages cheaper, which increased sugar consumption among kids.

VULNERABILITY TO CARBOHYDRATES

Because we modern humans consume so much starch and sugar, we take in literally hundreds of times more glucose than our prehistoric ancestors did. This extra glucose doesn't seem to affect some people. They eat the same food as everyone else and stay slim and healthy. However, a lot of us don't handle all this glucose so well. It makes us fat and diabetic, increases our risk of heart disease, brings on gout, and causes low testosterone in men and infertility in women.

Why are some more vulnerable than others to the toxic effects of a starchy, sugary diet? The problem is insulin resistance. People with insulin resistance produce as much as six times the normal amounts of insulin when they eat carbohydrates. This isn't good. Forcing the beta cells to produce such large amounts of insulin can cause those cells to virtually wear out from overuse. When insulin production can't keep up with demand, blood glucose levels rise, which is when doctors diagnose adult-onset, or type 2, diabetes. (Note: This kind of diabetes is different from the kind that affects children, which is called juvenile, or type 1, diabetes. Kids with type 1 diabetes remain sensitive to insulin, but due to an immune response to an infection that damages their beta cells, they produce *lower* than normal amounts.)

Although insulin resistance often leads to diabetes, most people with insulin resistance manage to escape it—they continue making enough insulin to keep their blood glucose levels down. You might ask: if more insulin is what it takes to keep your blood sugar down and you don't have diabetes, what's the problem? The problem is that while your muscles might be unresponsive to insulin's effects, other parts of your body remain sensitive to it. Too much insulin overstimulates these systems, and that causes all kinds of trouble, including:

Obesity. As the body's main calorie-storing hormone, insulin converts calories into fat and stores them in your fat cells. Too much insulin promotes fat buildup, particularly in your abdomen, which is why you see so many potbellies these days. Increased abdominal girth is such a reliable sign that your body is producing too much insulin that the American Heart Association recommends using it as a guide to treatment.

High blood cholesterol. Insulin resistance does something tricky to your blood cholesterol level. It raises the number of cholesterol *particles* in your blood without increasing the actual *amount* of cholesterol. How can it do this? Cholesterol travels through your bloodstream in packets, or particles, each of which contains thousands of cholesterol molecules. Insulin resistance increases the number of those packets. However, each packet contains fewer cholesterol molecules. Thus, your cholesterol level might be normal, but the number of cholesterol particles in your blood is increased. It turns out that the number of cholesterol particles predicts your risk of heart attack better than the amount of cholesterol does.

High blood triglyceride. Insulin, combined with a diet high in carbohydrates, causes your liver to produce a type of fat called triglyceride, which is secreted into your bloodstream. Although triglyceride doesn't damage blood vessels, high levels of it lower the concentrations of so-called good cholesterol in your blood. Good cholesterol actually removes cholesterol from your arteries. High levels of it protect you from blood vessel disease; low levels increase your risk.

Increased blood pressure. Excessive insulin reduces salt excretion by your kidneys and constricts blood vessels, which raises blood pressure.

Excess testosterone in women. Insulin prods the ovaries to secrete testosterone—the so-called male hormone. Too much testosterone causes unwanted facial and body hair, thinning of scalp hair, and acne.

Ovulation problems. Insulin resistance can impair ovulation, trigger irregular periods, and cause cysts to accumulate in the ovaries. This often leads to polycystic ovary syndrome (PCOS), America's number one cause of infertility.

Reduced testosterone in men. High insulin levels cause men's testicles to secrete *less* testosterone—the opposite of what it does to women's ovaries. Testosterone deficiency reduces muscle mass, vitality, and sex drive in men.

A NEW RISK FACTOR FOR HEART DISEASE

The leading cause of death in both men and women in industrialized nations is cholesterol buildup in the arteries to the heart, the *coronary arteries*. For years, doctors recognized four risk factors for coronary artery disease:

1. Cigarette smoking
2. Imbalance between good and bad blood cholesterol levels
3. High blood pressure
4. Diabetes

Thanks to better control of these risk factors, fewer of us are dying of heart disease compared to forty years ago. However, doctors now recognize another risk factor for coronary artery disease— insulin resistance. In the last forty years, as doctors learned to deal with other risk factors, the number of Americans with insulin resistance skyrocketed, negating much of the progress that has been made against heart disease. Insulin resistance does a quadruple whammy on the risk factors; it raises the number of cholesterol particles in your blood, lowers good cholesterol, increases blood pressure, and raises the risk of diabetes. The number of people with insulin resistance is rising so fast that some scientists are saying that younger people may end up living shorter lives than their parents.

THE CARBOHYDRATE–OVARY CONNECTION

In 1993, insulin resistance was among the furthest things from the minds of fertility specialists (doctors who specialize in helping women get pregnant). Insulin-related issues were the concern of doctors who treated diabetics. Fertility specialists had no idea that insulin had anything to do with the ovaries. Then came one of the most amazingly serendipitous discoveries in the history of medicine.

By far, the most common cause of infertility in the United States and other industiralized countries is polycystic ovary syndrome (PCOS), with an estimated 18 percent of women— and 28 percent of overweight women—having PCOS. Women with PCOS suffer from various combinations of obesity, unwanted body hair, acne, menstrual difficulties, and infertility. Incredibly, most girls and women who have PCOS are unaware they have it. PCOS can be devastating to women's lives. It damages self-esteem in teenage girls and derails women's dreams of having children. Sociologists Celia Kitzinger and Jo Willmott, who studied the social and psychological impact of PCOS on women, called it "a thief of womanhood."

In 1993, the pharmaceutical company Bristol-Myers Squibb began marketing a new medication for treating diabetes called metformin. Previous diabetes drugs had reduced blood sugar by raising insulin levels. Metformin works by reducing the body's need for insulin. It actually *lowers* insulin levels. Soon after metformin came on the market, doctors began noticing cases of women with PCOS who also happened to have diabetes and became pregnant soon after taking it. At first, doctors thought it was coincidental, but some were impressed enough to submit case reports to medical journals for publication. It soon became apparent that these weren't isolated instances. Metformin not only restores normal ovulation and fertility in women with PCOS but also reduces the belly fat, stray body hair, and acne that often accompany the condition.

Before metformin came on the market, scientists were unaware of any connections between PCOS and insulin. The discovery that metformin can reverse PCOS sent scientists rushing to the laboratory to measure insulin resistance in these women. They found that, indeed, most women with PCOS have insulin resistance. This was a revolutionary discovery. Previously, doctors had thought PCOS was a genetic defect confined to the ovaries. Although it's true that some women are genetically predisposed to PCOS, insulin resistance brings it on. The culprit is not just insulin; it's *excessive* insulin. Too much insulin causes the ovaries to overproduce testosterone, which brings on the stray body hair and acne and interferes with egg maturation by the ovaries. In many women with PCOS, periods become irregular, unreleased eggs turn into cysts, and it becomes increasingly difficult to get pregnant.

The discovery that insulin resistance causes PCOS also explains why so many PCOS sufferers are overweight. Excessive insulin promotes abdominal fat buildup. Although some women with PCOS are not overweight, they still tend to accumulate fat in their abdomen. Using special scans to measure body fat in various parts of the body, scientists found that women with PCOS who are not overweight still have more than normal amounts of fat in their abdomen relative to the rest of their body.

Whereas high insulin levels bring on PCOS, anything that lowers insulin levels—cutting carbohydrates, exercising, or taking medications that reduce insulin needs—can reverse it.

ERECTILE DYSFUNCTION AND LOW TESTOSTERONE

In April 1998, doctors' phones were ringing off the hook. Viagra had come on the market for treating erectile dysfunction, or E.D. Although difficulty attaining an erection is common among middle-aged and older males, most men were hesitant to complain about it to their doctors, perhaps figuring that a dwindling sex life was an inevitable part of aging. The fact that a pill could restore their erections sent them a clear message that E.D. was a treatable medical condition. Viagra opened up a new field in medicine—men's sexual health. Men began viewing waning sexual function as a correctible body chemistry imbalance rather than an inevitable effect of aging. They became open to the idea that improving their body chemistry could restore an active sex life.

There are two types of sexual impairment in men. One is difficulty attaining an erection despite a healthy desire for sex; the other is waning desire. It turns out that insulin resistance worsens both of these problems. Researchers have reported that as many as 79 percent of men with such difficulties have insulin resistance.

Normally, sexual arousal triggers the penile arteries to open and allow blood to rush in, which produces an erection. The usual cause of E.D. is a failure of those arteries to dilate fully. Drugs such as Viagra help the penile arteries open wider in response to sexual stimuli. Insulin resistance reduces the ability of those arteries to fully open. Studies show that reducing insulin resistance with proper diet and exercise can restore normal erections.

The other category of reduced sexual activity that comes with aging is loss of interest in sex. In the past, men attributed waning sex drive to fatigue or boredom. In fact, reduced levels of testosterone, a hormone that increases sexual desire, causes much of the decline. Doctors often treat men who have low testosterone with testosterone supplements, which often restore their interest in sex. Insulin resistance inhibits testosterone production by the testicles; alleviating insulin resistance increases testosterone levels, and often restores men's libido. Although testosterone levels normally decline with age, many men maintain sexual function into their eighties.

AN UNFORESEEN EPIDEMIC

So why aren't we as healthy as scientists forty years ago thought we were going to be? We've been blindsided by an epidemic of insulin resistance. The problem is that until this epidemic was upon us, doctors didn't know there was such a thing as insulin resistance. Measuring the body's responsiveness to insulin is a complicated procedure that can only be done in specialized laboratories. It wasn't until the 2000s that researchers figured out how to detect insulin resistance and discovered how widespread it is. In the past decade, practicing doctors have learned how to diagnose insulin resistance by looking for signs of its effects. In fact, with a tape measure and a phone call to your doctor, you can probably diagnose it yourself. The next chapter will show you how.

2

HOW TO TELL WHETHER YOU ARE INSULIN RESISTANT

Scientists haven't come up with an easy way to measure insulin resistance. You might think that you could diagnose it by just giving someone insulin and seeing how much it lowers blood glucose. The problem for patients is that low blood sugar is uncomfortable and even dangerous. Scientists get around this by infusing insulin into one vein and glucose into another and measuring blood levels every few minutes for several hours. This is called a "glucose clamp" test. Don't expect your doctor to do this test, however; it's only done in specialized research laboratories. Another way to diagnose insulin resistance is to measure the levels of insulin in your blood. Higher-than-normal insulin levels suggest that you have insulin resistance. However, because insulin leaves the bloodstream so fast, it's difficult to tell how much your beta cells are producing by measuring blood levels.

Although it's difficult to measure insulin resistance directly, doctors have learned to detect it by looking for signs of its effects on the body. The more of the following signs you have, the higher your likelihood is of being insulin resistant. If you have three or more of these signs, doctors would say you have metabolic syndrome, in which case, chances are eight in ten that you have insulin resistance. Notice that these aren't just signs of a problem, they are also problems themselves. Let's take a closer look.

A tendency to store fat in the abdomen. In addition to promoting weight gain, insulin resistance redistributes fat from your hips and thighs to your abdomen—your belly gets bigger relative to your buttocks and thighs. A good way to tell whether you have insulin resistance is to simply wrap a measuring tape around your abdomen. Researchers have established criteria for diagnosing insulin resistance by correlating abdominal girth with glucose clamp tests to measure insulin sensitivity. If the circumference of your abdomen exceeds the limits below, odds are you're insulin resistant. (Remember, pants size doesn't count. You need to wrap a measuring tape around your abdomen at the level of your navel.)

Men: *40 inches (102 cm) or more (Asian-American men, 35 inches [89 cm] or more)*
Women: *35 inches (89 cm) or more (Asian-American women, 32 inches [81.3 cm] or more)*

Although most insulin-resistant folks have larger-than-normal abdomens, some don't. However, these individuals often have more fat in their abdomens relative to their buttocks and thighs. You can tell whether you fit this pattern by dividing your abdominal girth by the circumference of your hips, measured around the plumpest part of your buttocks—the waist-to-hip ratio, as doctors call it. A waist-to-hip ratio greater than 80 percent for females—and 95 percent for males—usually means you are insulin resistant.

You don't always need a tape measure to determine whether a person has insulin resistance; you can often tell at a glance. Doctors describe folks who carry their weight in the upper half of the body as "apple-shaped," and those who carry their weight around the thighs and buttocks as "pear-shaped." They have observed that being apple-shaped carries a greater risk of diabetes and heart disease than being pear-shaped.

Notice that fat patterns differ between Asians and non-Asians. Asians develop insulin resistance with less enlargement of abdominal girth than non-Asians do.

Fat patterns also differ between men and women. Estrogen, the so-called female hormone, does the opposite of insulin, shifting fat away from the abdomen to the buttocks and thighs. Estrogen gives women their distinctive shape—narrow waist and full hips. As women age, these levels gradually dwindle and then drop off precipitously at menopause. Dwindling estrogen levels, combined with insulin resistance, bring on the dreaded midlife spread, which increases with age.

High blood levels of triglyceride. Insulin resistance, combined with a diet high in carbohydrates, activates pathways in your liver that convert excess glucose into a type of fat called triglyceride. High blood levels of triglyceride are a good indicator of insulin resistance. You can probably find out what your triglyceride level is by calling your doctor's office. A triglyceride level higher than

150 if you haven't eaten for 12 hours, or higher than 175 if you have, suggests that you have insulin resistance.

One problem with using triglyceride measurements to diagnose insulin resistance is that triglyceride levels fluctuate rapidly with changes in your eating and exercise activities. A couple of days of increased exercise and avoidance of starch and sugar can reduce your levels significantly. The best time to measure your triglyceride level is when you haven't been restricting carbohydrates or exercising more than usual.

Low levels of "good cholesterol." As you've probably heard, cholesterol can build up in your arteries and cause blockages. Cholesterol circulates in your blood in two forms: LDL, nicknamed bad cholesterol, and HDL, called good cholesterol. The higher your LDL levels, the higher your chances of developing cholesterol buildup in your arteries. On the other hand, HDL helps remove cholesterol from your arteries. The higher your good cholesterol, the less likely you are to have blood vessel problems.

High levels of triglyceride deplete HDL. Indeed, the usual cause of low HDL is high blood triglyceride. However, although triglyceride levels fluctuate a lot from day to day, HDL levels change more slowly. Thus, low HDL is a more stable indicator of insulin resistance. Doctors usually measure HDL when they check cholesterol. Women normally have higher HDL levels than men do. An HDL level lower than 50 for women or 40 for men suggests insulin resistance.

Slightly increased blood pressure. Insulin resistance triggers reflexes in your kidneys and blood vessels that raise your blood pressure *a little*; insulin resistance alone won't raise your blood pressure to harmfully high levels. Healthy adults usually have blood pressure readings of 120/80 or less. Readings higher than 130/85 suggest insulin resistance even if they don't exceed 140/90, the level most doctors consider high.

Increased blood glucose level. If you have insulin resistance, your beta cells compensate by secreting more insulin and your glucose levels usually stay in a safe range. But even though you don't have what doctors would call diabetes, your levels are likely to be slightly higher than average. Your fasting blood glucose level, when you haven't eaten for 12 hours, should normally be less than 100. Readings between 100 and 125 don't mean you have diabetes, but they are suggestive of insulin resistance.

The problem with measuring blood glucose levels is that readings vary according to your food consumption and exercise in the previous day or two. Doctors now have a measurement called the A1C test, which is unaffected by short-term changes in diet and exercise. Here's how it works: Each time your blood sugar rises, it puts a tiny coating of glucose on your red blood cells, which stays there for the life of the cells—about three months. The A1C test measures this glucose and tells you what your average blood sugar has been for the previous three months. Normally, your A1C level should be less than 6.0. A level of 6.5 or higher usually means you have diabetes. A "borderline" level, between 6.0 and 6.5, suggests insulin resistance. (Note: Because the A1C test isn't affected by what you ate or how much you exercised in the previous day or two, you don't need to fast before taking it.)

OTHER WAYS TO TELL

The problem with looking for signs of metabolic syndrome to detect insulin resistance is that a lot of people who have insulin resistance don't show those signs. About a third of individuals with insulin resistance diagnosed by a glucose clamp test do not qualify as having metabolic syndrome. One reason is that it takes years for signs of metabolic syndrome to develop. Individuals who have obvious evidence of it in midlife may show no signs of it in their youth. Moreover, genes affect how insulin resistance manifests itself. Some people are genetically more prone to obesity, high blood pressure, high triglyceride, and high blood sugar, regardless of insulin resistance.

PCOS—A Sure Sign of Insulin Resistance

If you have polycystic ovary syndrome (PCOS), you are virtually certain to be insulin resistant even if you have no signs of metabolic syndrome. Doctors diagnose PCOS by looking for evidence of excessive testosterone secretion and disturbed egg production by the ovaries. If you have any two of the following three signs, you are likely to have PCOS:

- Late, irregular, or unusually heavy periods, or blood tests indicating that you are not ovulating regularly.
- Evidence of testosterone excess. This includes adult acne, excessive body hair with thinning scalp hair, or blood tests showing higher-than-normal levels of testosterone.
- More than ten cysts in your ovaries detected by ultrasound.

Even if you don't have PCOS, having even one of these signs increases the likelihood that you are insulin resistant. Insulin resistance can bring on acne, increased body hair, thinning scalp hair, menstrual irregularities, and reduced fertility alone or in combination. On the positive side, reducing insulin resistance has been shown to improve all of these conditions.

The Fogginess of Low Blood Sugar

A common symptom of insulin resistance is what doctors call reactive hypoglycemia, or low blood sugar. Normally, when you eat carbohydrates, your beta cells respond to rising blood glucose by secreting exactly the right amount of insulin to ease it back down. However, if you have insulin resistance, your beta cells react to rising blood sugar by secreting more-than-normal amounts of insulin, sometimes driving blood sugar down too fast. Three or four hours after eating a starchy meal, you may feel shaky, have trouble concentrating, and become voraciously hungry—symptoms that are promptly relieved by eating. In one experiment, researchers injected subjects with insulin to lower their blood sugar levels to the point of causing hypoglycemia, and then observed the kinds of foods they chose to eat. Low blood sugar gave them a preference for starchy, sugary snacks—foods that boost blood sugar fast, but ironically are the kinds that cause reactive hypoglycemia in the first place.

Reactive hypoglycemia can reduce your efficiency at performing mental work. Low blood sugar impairs what psychologists call working memory—the ability to hold a thought in mind long enough to carry out a response. A good example of someone using working memory is a computer programmer trying to hold a sequence of software commands in mind long enough to enter them into a computer. Hypoglycemia reduces efficiency in performing such tasks.

Driven by Adrenaline

Your nervous system responds to falling blood sugar by secreting adrenaline, which raises your blood sugar. Adrenaline is the "fight-or-flight" hormone. It enhances physical performance. Mother Nature gave us adrenaline to help us deal with dangers of the physical kind—saber-toothed tigers and such. Adrenaline increases your heart rate, tenses your muscles, quickens your breathing, and creates a feeling of uneasiness, as if to heighten your awareness of danger. Though these surges can prepare you for physical exertion, if you're sitting at a desk, all they do is jangle your nerves. By the end of the day, alternating restlessness and fatigue caused by fluctuating blood sugar and adrenaline levels can leave you feeling exhausted and out of sorts.

The cure for this problem? For years, even before they learned about insulin resistance, doctors knew that reducing starch and sugar at meals prevents reactive hypoglycemia later. Avoiding rapidly digestible carbohydrates prevents the insulin overshoot that drives blood sugar down so fast.

Of course, a lot of things can cause anxiety, poor concentration, and fatigue. However, if you have these symptoms, consider the possibility of reactive hypoglycemia.

3

WHAT CAUSES INSULIN RESISTANCE?

If insulin resistance brings on all of these problems, what causes it? It helps to understand that there are two kinds—a normal kind that occurs after you eat a starchy meal and goes away in a few hours, and an abnormal kind that sticks around for weeks and brings on problems such as belly fat, diabetes, and polycystic ovary syndrome (PCOS). The problem is that too much of the normal kind brings on the abnormal kind. Here's what happens.

DEALING WITH A CARB-FILLED MEAL

One of insulin's jobs is to open the gates on the surface of your muscle cells that allow glucose to pass into them. This gives the cells a way to control the amount of glucose that enters them. If your muscle cells have all the glucose they need, they stop responding to insulin—they "lock" the gates. This kind of insulin resistance happens to all of us when we eat more carbohydrates than we burn off with physical activity. This is a good thing because glucose draws water into cells. Too much glucose in your cells would cause them to literally swell up and burst.

What happens to the leftover glucose? That's what fat is for. Fat is made up of specialized cells designed to store calories. Your fat cells keep responding to insulin after your muscles stop doing so. If you have more glucose in your bloodstream than your muscles need, insulin converts it to fat and pushes it into your fat cells. Make no mistake: You don't have to eat fat to get fat. Insulin turns carbs into fat. That potato you ate last night? Insulin turned it into lard, and it's now resting on your thighs.

But glucose isn't the only substance insulin pushes into your fat cells. As your body's main calorie-storing hormone, insulin forces fuel from all three kinds of food—fat, protein, and carbohydrates—into your fuel tank. When you consume more carbs than your muscles burn off, insulin changes *everything you eat* into fat. This kind of insulin resistance might be normal for *us,* but not for a cave dweller. Prehistoric humans didn't have enough carbohydrates in their diet to have to deal with extra glucose.

WHEN YOUR FUEL TANK RUNS OVER

The after-meal kind of insulin resistance happens to all of us when we eat more carbs than we need to replace the ones we've burned off. Now let's talk about the abnormal kind—the kind that sticks around for weeks and brings on problems such as belly fat, diabetes, and PCOS.

Okay, you ate too many carbs. A few hours have passed and all that leftover glucose has turned into fat. You gained a little weight, but at least you got the excess glucose out of your blood. Your insulin levels have come back down, and now you have a fresh start. As long as you don't do the same thing at the next meal—eat more carbs than you burn off—your muscle cells will use up the glucose in them and start responding to insulin again. Increased responsiveness to insulin means you won't have to produce a lot of insulin to handle whatever carbohydrates you eat. Lower insulin levels will allow your fat cells to release calories back into your system. That's what fat cells are for—to store and release fuel to provide energy between meals.

But what if you eat more carbohydrates than your muscles burn off, meal after meal, day after day? What if your muscles are continually shutting off to insulin and your beta cells are repeatedly having to make more insulin than normal and pushing more calories into your fat cells? There's a limit to the amount of fuel your fat cells can store. What happens when they can't hold any more fuel? This happens a lot—in fact, we're in an epidemic of this happening. When insulin tries to force fuel into fat cells that can't hold any more, fuel starts leaking out as fast as it goes in. It's like trying to put gas in your car when the tank is full: it spills out and makes a big mess.

THE FATTY ACID FLOOD

When fuel spills out of your fat cells, it doesn't revert back to the form that it arrived in—it leaves as *fatty acid*, a breakdown product of fat. When your fat cells overflow, they flood your whole system with fatty acid, and that causes trouble. Fatty acid infiltrates every cell of your body, which causes them to function less efficiently. They lose responsiveness to a number of hormones, and one of those hormones is insulin. In other words, fatty acid overflow worsens insulin resistance.

Do you see a problem here? Now you have a vicious cycle. High insulin levels are what caused your system to be flooded with fatty acids in the first place. Now those fatty acids are making you even more insulin resistant and raising your insulin levels even more. This is when your metabolism falls off a cliff. Fatty acids make your muscle cells more resistant to insulin than ever. You may need five or six times the normal amount of insulin to handle the carbohydrates you eat. This kind of insulin resistance doesn't go away in a few hours like the normal, after-meal kind does. It lingers for weeks. When you're in this state and you get anywhere near a carbohydrate, your insulin levels skyrocket, driving more fuel into your fat cells, wearing out your beta cells, and messing up your sex hormones.

Fat cell overflow also brings on belly fat. Your body uses the fat depots in your abdomen as a sort of garbage dump. Your abdomen takes up fat the rest of your body can't hold, which is why an increased abdominal girth is a good indicator of insulin resistance.

HOW INSULIN RESISTANCE MAKES YOU FAT

No one needs to be convinced that we have an obesity problem. Look around you. The percentage of overweight Americans has doubled in fifty years. Two-thirds are overweight; a third are obese—30 pounds (13.7 kg) or more overweight. This epidemic has spread to other industrialized nations as Europe and Asia are also seeing obesity rates skyrocket. However, this weight gain isn't evenly distributed in the population. For example, the slimmer half of the population is only about 10 pounds (4.5 kg) heavier than the slimmer half was fifty years ago, the heavier half is 30 pounds (13.7 kg) heavier. The heaviest 10 percent are a whopping *60* pounds (27.2 kg) heavier than the heaviest 10 percent was fifty years ago. It seems that whatever caused us to gain weight in the last fifty years triggered a vicious cycle in some of us that resulted in extreme weight gain.

What happened to make so many of us overweight, and why, for some folks, does gaining weight seen to generate a vicious cycle of even more weight gain? You can't blame it on genetics; genes take thousands of years to change. Something we're doing or not doing is making us all gain weight and causing some of us to become dangerously fat. Of course, the usual explanation is lack of willpower, but why would so many of us suddenly lose our willpower? Every day you see people who display remarkable discipline in other aspects of their lives yet still have trouble with their weight. The lack-of-willpower explanation just doesn't make sense.

WHY WILLPOWER DOESN'T WORK

Remember when you were a kid and you tried to see how long you could hold your breath? It was easy at first, but after 30 seconds or so your body told you, in no uncertain terms, that it was time to breathe. Carbon dioxide accumulated in your system, stimulated breathing centers in your brain, and made you breathe no matter how hard you tried not to. You quickly learned that you can't resist your body's demands.

The same thing happens when you try to lose weight by just trying to eat less. As reasonable as it sounds, it rarely works. Just as chemical reactions in your body determine how much air you breathe, others control how much food you eat, and it's almost impossible to resist them. However, that doesn't mean you can't lose weight. You just need to get your body chemistry working for you rather than against you. If you understand what kind of chemical reactions are going on in your body that are making you gain weight, you will find that it's not hard to reverse them.

Internal Starvation

You probably have at least a month's worth of fuel stored up as fat. Ask yourself this: With all that extra fuel, why is it that a few hours after eating a meal you're hungry again? Why doesn't your body just use the fuel stored up in your fat to keep you from getting hungry?

If you're like most folks having trouble with their weight, the problem is too much insulin. Insulin activates enzymes that push calories into your fat cells and inhibit the ones that transport them out. Too much insulin in your system pushes fuel into your fat cells and locks it in. Fuel can't go to your muscles to be used for energy or your brain to quell your hunger. Consequently, a couple of hours after eating, your brain senses you're running out of fuel, and you're hungry again. Scientists call this *internal starvation*. Your fat stores act like a giant tumor—they keep growing while the rest of your body starves.

Where does the excess insulin come from? You already know the answer. You don't need insulin to handle the fat and protein in your diet, you only need it to handle carbohydrates. If you eat a lot of carbohydrates, you make a lot of insulin. Does that mean you'll get fat if you eat carbohydrates? Not necessarily. Your body has ways of putting the brakes on fat storage.

Appetite-Control Hormones

It turns out that Mother Nature doesn't want you to be fat any more than you do. Normally, when you eat enough food to replenish the calories you've burned off, your body produces hormones that travel to the appetite-control centers of your brain and interact with these centers to quell your hunger. An example of such a hormone is *leptin*, which is produced by your fat cells. Leptin travels through your bloodstream to your brain and suppresses hunger. It helps keep you from accumulating too much fat. The more fat you store, the more leptin you produce and the less you should want to eat—that is, if your appetite-control centers are working right.

Scientists have discovered several appetite-control hormones. Some come from the stomach and intestines and respond to the amount of food you eat during a meal. Some, such as leptin, come from your fat cells and respond to the amount of fat you store up. Scientists can actually reduce people's food intake by administering these hormones. But here's the problem: most obese individuals' appetite-control centers are resistant to the effects of these hormones. Their fat cells make plenty of leptin, for example, but the appetite-control centers in their brain don't respond to it the way they should.

Why would the appetite-control centers in your brain stop working just when you need them the most—when you're overweight? Remember the fatty acid flood? In addition to infiltrating your muscle cells and making them more resistant to insulin, fatty acids accumulate in the appetite-control centers of your brain, which reduce their responsiveness to hormones such as leptin. You end up eating more than you need—not because you lack willpower but because the hunger-control centers in your brain aren't functioning properly.

Let's go through that sequence of events again. If you consume more carbohydrates than your muscles burn off, your blood glucose level rises and the beta cells of your pancreas produce more insulin to try to get your glucose level down. Excessive insulin pushes calories into your fat cells and locks it in so fuel can't get to the hunger-control centers in your brain—internal starvation. That's okay for a meal or two, but if you keep consuming more carbs than you burn off and insulin keeps driving fuel into your fat cells, at some point those cells can't hold any more fuel and fatty acid starts spilling into your bloodstream.

That's when the vicious cycle begins. Fatty acid accumulates in your muscle cells, making them even more resistant to insulin, and in the appetite-control centers of your brain, making them less responsive to your appetite-control hormones. Just when you need your hunger-suppressing hormones the most—when you store so much fuel that your fat cells are spilling fatty acids into your bloodstream—the appetite-control centers in your brain decide to go on strike. Your weight spirals out of control—not because you lack willpower, but because your body chemistry has fallen out of whack.

And at the root of it all is *too much insulin*.

The Couch Potato Trap

When you gain weight, there's usually another vicious cycle at work. As everyone knows, exercise helps you control your weight. It not only burns calories, but it also sensitizes your muscles to insulin—it counteracts insulin resistance. The problem is that when you gain weight, physical activity takes more effort, so you tend to be less active. Less exercise makes you gain even more weight, which makes exercise even harder. Normally, your appetite-control centers should adjust to reduced physical activity and curb your appetite. However, if you're insulin resistant, lack of exercise causes you to produce more insulin, which raises your fatty acid levels even more, guaranteeing that your appetite-control centers will continue to malfunction. They don't adjust to your sedentary behavior. You end up being as hungry as you were when you were more physically active.

REVERSING THE VICIOUS CYCLE

You can turn the vicious cycle of weight gain into a virtuous cycle of weight loss by reducing the insulin that feeds the vicious cycle. Lower insulin levels allow the fuel from meals to go to your brain to satisfy your hunger instead of to your fat stores. When insulin stops pushing fuel into your fat cells, you stop spilling fatty acids into your bloodstream. Your muscles use up the fatty acids in them and start responding to insulin again. Eventually, fatty acids clear out of the appetite-control centers of your brain, allowing these centers to regain their ability to balance your food intake with your energy expenditure. Part II of this book will show you how to restore your body's responsiveness to insulin and reduce those insulin levels that perpetuate the vicious cycle.

4 A MODERN EPIDEMIC

We all eat more carbohydrates than our systems were designed to handle. Why then do only some of us develop problems like abdominal obesity, diabetes, and polycystic ovary syndrome (PCOS)? If insulin resistance is the problem, then why do only some of us get it? Genetics play a role. Having a family history of type 2 diabetes or PCOS increases the likelihood of developing insulin resistance. Scientists have found differences in the *mitochondria*—tiny fuel-burning units—in the muscle cells of family members of adult-onset diabetics years before they become overweight or develop diabetes.

Another problem is that some people have genetically smaller "gas tanks" than others do. Their fat cells can't store as much fat. As soon as they gain a few extra pounds, they start spilling fatty acid into their bloodstream. They might not even be overweight. Using special scans to measure body fat, scientists have found that people who have insulin resistance but are not overweight usually have more than normal amounts of fat in their abdomen relative to the rest of their body.

Genes also influence how women's ovaries respond to insulin. Not all women who over-produce insulin secrete excess testosterone or develop PCOS. In addition, genes affect the tendency to develop acne or excess hair growth in response to testosterone.

Although genetics matter, keep in mind that insulin resistance was much less common as recently as forty years ago. Our genes didn't change. Something we're doing or not doing has triggered an epidemic of insulin resistance.

THE INDUSTRIAL REVOLUTION

Until the 1900s, most people spent their days doing physical work. The majority lived on farms. Cars and buses hadn't been invented, and walking was the main form of transportation. Then came what historians call the Industrial Revolution. In the last half of the nineteenth century, mechanization began to change the workplace. Eventually, much of the physical exertion of work was taken over by machines. Mechanized farm equipment reduced the need for farm labor. The largest population shift in the history of the United States occurred during the first half of the twentieth century, when the children of farmers moved to towns and cities and took up less physically demanding occupations.

Mechanization also changed the way we get around. Cars, buses, trains, and elevators took over the job of moving us from place to place. In the nineteenth century, people typically walked several miles (kilometers) a day. Now we go days without walking more than a couple hundred feet (60 m).

In the last forty years, computerization has made office work even more sedentary than it was. Television screens and computer terminals have a mesmerizing effect that freezes movement. Scientists have found that the more time people spend working on a computer or watching television, the higher their risk of obesity and diabetes. Along with mechanization of work and transportation came a steady increase in the average body weight. As people became more sedentary, doctors started seeing more adults with diabetes. They thought it curious that unlike children with diabetes, who were usually underweight, adult-onset diabetics were usually overweight.

The main reason insulin resistance is more common now than it was in the nineteenth century is that we are less physically active. Regular exercise is 100 percent effective at relieving insulin resistance. It prevents obesity and diabetes, restores fertility in women with PCOS, and improves sexual function and vitality in men. However, if you are riding to work in a car or bus, sitting in front of a computer all day, watching television at night, and not getting regular exercise, you are setting yourself up for insulin resistance.

The good news is that you don't have to sweat and strain to restore your body's sensitivity to insulin. The next chapter will show you how to reverse insulin resistance with a kind of exercise that even couch potatoes can do. You will see that the types of muscle activity most effective at eliminating insulin resistance are, by their nature, the easiest to do.

THE OBESITY EPIDEMIC

Although obesity and diabetes rates rose during the industrial revolution, the percentage of Americans who had these conditions remained relatively constant until the 1970s, when the numbers suddenly shot up. Between 1970 and 2000, the percentage of Americans who were obese—30 pounds (13.7 kg) overweight or more—doubled. The incidence of diabetes tripled. What happened?

Beyond physical inactivity, what makes us insulin resistant is a diet high in starch and sugar. After the Great Depression and World War II, most people considered it a privilege to be able to eat eggs, meat, and dairy products. For the first time in history, agricultural mass production, refrigeration, and rapid transportation made fresh produce available and affordable. People remembered the Great Depression and war years, when many suffered from iron, protein, and vitamin deficiencies caused by lack of adequate nutrition. The ability to enjoy abundant fresh produce, which prevented such problems, was considered a blessing. Americans were well fed in the 1950s and '60s, yet obesity and diabetes were much less common than they are today.

The Great Cholesterol Experiment

Around 1970, something happened that dampened the enthusiasm for eggs, meat, and dairy products. This is when the FDA and medical organizations concerned about the rising incidence of heart disease began recommending reduced consumption of cholesterol-containing foods. The theory, *since disproved*, was that reducing the cholesterol consumed from food would reduce the cholesterol in the blood and prevent cholesterol buildup in the arteries.

Scientists later learned that most of the cholesterol in people's blood does not come from the cholesterol in food. In fact, the liver makes it. Cutting cholesterol in the diet doesn't lower blood cholesterol. Actually, cholesterol is hard to digest. Most of it passes through your intestinal tract and out in the stool. Your liver regulates the amount of cholesterol in your blood. If you eat less cholesterol, your liver makes more of it; if you eat more, it makes less.

Nevertheless, we got the message that dietary cholesterol was bad and did what we were told despite insufficient evidence that cutting cholesterol would do any good. According to U.S. Department of Agriculture (USDA) statistics, average red meat consumption per person fell by 16 percent between 1970 and 1997. Egg consumption fell by 23 percent, and milk fat consumption fell by 52 percent.

Of course, if you eat less of one kind of food, you usually end up eating more of another. When Americans started eating fewer eggs and dairy products and less meat, they began to consume more carbohydrates, but not the natural kind found in fresh fruit and vegetables. They started eating more refined carbohydrates—a *lot* more. USDA statistics show that by 1997, Americans were eating 48 percent more flour, 186 percent more rice, and 131 percent more frozen potato products (mainly French fries) than they did in 1970.

America's largest source of starch, by far, is wheat. The graph in Figure 1 (see page 30) compares the average wheat consumption per person from 1960 to 2000 with the percentage of people who were 30 pounds (13.7 kg) or more overweight. You can see that as soon as wheat

Figure 1: Obesity Rate versus Wheat Consumption (pounds per person, 1961–2000)

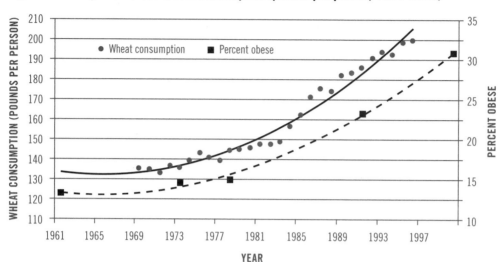

Source: Rob Thompson, M.D.

consumption started rising in the 1970s, the obesity rate did the same. (It is understandable why cardiologist William Davis, M.D., author of *Wheat Belly,* blames the obesity and diabetes epidemics on wheat consumption alone.)

Although mechanization of the workplace and motorized transportation set the stage for our current epidemic of insulin resistance, the increased consumption of starch and sugar that has occurred since the 1970s pushed us over the edge. If you consider that modern humans consume hundreds of times more glucose in the form of rapidly digestible carbohydrates than their prehistoric ancestors did and significantly more than people forty years ago did, it's not surprising that more of us than ever are suffering from problems caused by insulin resistance. Studies show that people who consume more than average amounts of rapidly digestible carbohydrates—flour products, potatoes, rice, and sugary beverages—have increase rates of obesity, diabetes, gout, and PCOS. Indeed, the latest FDA guidelines represent a complete reversal of previous recommendations. Fat and cholesterol are no longer considered "nutrients of concern." The new guidelines recommend limiting consumption of refined carbohydrates.

PART II

THE SOLUTION FOR RECLAIMING A NORMAL METABOLISM

5

ACTIVATE YOUR SLOW-TWITCH MUSCLES

Insulin resistance is like an overflowing sink. To stop the flooding (of your body with insulin), you need to turn off the faucet (reduce the amount of glucose going into your system) and unplug the drain (restore your muscles' responsiveness to insulin). You can't get away with doing one; you need to do both. If you reduce your carbohydrate intake without sensitizing your muscles to insulin, then even small amounts of carbohydrates will drive up your insulin levels. If you restore your muscles' responsiveness to insulin but keep flooding your system with glucose, then your muscles will stop responding to insulin and your levels will skyrocket again.

If this sounds like the same old advice you've heard in the past—just eat less and exercise more—it isn't. This is not about cutting calories—*it's about reducing insulin levels.* The good news is that it isn't hard to do. In the past, folks did it without even trying. Thanks to recent research on the effects of various foods on insulin production, we know you don't need to deprive yourself of good food. You only need to avoid a few culprits that cause your body to produce unusually large amounts of insulin. And thanks to recent discoveries on how muscles respond to insulin, you don't have to huff and puff to restore their responsiveness to insulin. Exercising to relieve insulin resistance is a lot easier than trying to burn calories. You can reduce your body's insulin production to a fraction of what it was without going hungry or working out at a gym simply by combining what's called a *low-glycemic load* eating pattern, discussed in the next chapter, with activation of a type of muscle fiber scientists call a *slow-twitch* fiber.

THE *REAL* REASON EXERCISE WORKS

As a doctor, I can tell you that what changes people's lives is not diet, but exercise. Few people succeed in losing weight and keeping it off if they don't increase their activity level. Practicing doctors know this, but for years, this fact was not fully appreciated by scientists. They knew that it takes more exercise than most people think to burn calories. For example, you have to run 2 miles (3.2 km) to burn the calories you get from a single slice of bread. If you looked at exercise only as a way to burn calories, you'd think it wasn't very important.

Scientists now realize that the reason exercise works so well for losing weight and preventing diabetes is not because it burns calories, but because it eliminates insulin resistance. Exercise breaks up the metabolic logjam in your muscles that causes your system to be flooded with insulin every time you come near a carbohydrate.

Within minutes of starting a brisk walk, for example, your muscles start responding to insulin. If you walk for a half hour or so, they remain responsive for 24 to 48 hours. During that time, your body doesn't have to produce as much insulin as it did before, and the vicious cycle of insulin resistance reverses itself. Insulin stops pushing calories into your fat cells; fuel can get to your brain to satisfy your hunger and to your muscle cells to provide them with energy. All of this goes on for up to 48 hours after you exercise, even while you're sleeping. Nothing—not diet, not medications—relieves insulin resistance as quickly and as thoroughly as physical exercise.

THE MAGIC OF SLOW-TWITCH MUSCLE EXERCISE

Of course, you already know that exercise is good for you. The problem is that it's a lot of work, right? Here's the best news you've ever heard about exercise: Believe it or not, you have muscles in your body that *do not* get tired when you exercise them. If that sounds crazy, think about your breathing muscles—the ones in your chest that operate your lungs. How tired do you get from breathing? These muscles can work continuously without tiring because they're powered by a special type of muscle fiber called a slow-twitch fiber, which is full of tiny energy generators called mitochondria. Mitochondria use oxygen to restore the energy muscles use *as they are being used.* In contrast, muscle cells powered with the other kind of fiber—*fast-twitch* fibers—contain few mitochondria. Although they're good at operating temporarily without oxygen, they build up an oxygen "debt" when you use them, which must be repaid with rest. This debt is what causes muscles to fatigue.

It turns out that your breathing muscles aren't the only muscles in your body powered by slow-twitch fibers. They also power your walking muscles. That's right: *The muscles you use for walking do not tire out like other muscles.* Think about it. If you had to, you could walk for hours without stopping. You might get bored, your feet might get sore, but you could keep walking. What other exercise could you do for hours without stopping?

Although your breathing muscles comprise only a small portion of your total musculature, your walking muscles are another matter. They make up approximately 70 percent of your muscle mass. When you're walking, you might not feel like you're getting much exercise, but you really are. Walking a couple of miles (3.2 km) burns approximately 85 percent as many calories as running the same distance. The big difference is that walking is a lot easier than running. When scientists asked subjects to rate their effort level while performing various kinds of exercise, they found that of all the different kinds of physical activity people do, walking provides the most exercise with least amount of *perceived* exertion.

Remember those little energy generators in your slow-twitch muscles—the mitochondria? Your walking muscles contain most of the mitochondria in your body. It turns out that mitochondria are what determine your muscles' responsiveness to insulin. In other words, the muscles you need to exercise to relieve insulin resistance are exactly the ones that require the least amount of effort. Scientists took tissue samples from various muscles of subjects with and without insulin resistance and measured the enzymes involved in glucose metabolism. They found a deficiency of these enzymes in subjects with insulin resistance, but only in their leg muscles. It seems that insulin resistance is a disease of the legs, curable by walking.

Different Exercises Provide Different Benefits

What do you want from exercise? To be able to lift heavy objects? To win foot races? Probably what you want is to lose weight, look good, and stay healthy. Different kinds of exercise provide different benefits. If strengthening muscles is what you want, you need to strain them against resistance. A typical muscle-strengthening routine would be to lift a weight ten or twelve times in a row with the last repetition being against maximal resistance—as much as you can lift. Building endurance requires a different approach. How far you can run has little to do with muscle strength. It's determined by how much blood your heart can pump, which, in turn, is a matter of how fast your heart can beat, and how much blood it can pump with each beat—so-called "stroke volume." Although endurance training doesn't increase your maximal heart rate, it does increase your stroke volume. Building endurance requires you to get your heart pumping fast and keep it that way for 15 to 20 minutes. A typical routine would be to run a couple of miles (3.2 km) three or four times a week.

However, if what you want from exercise is to lose weight, prevent diabetes, and reduce your risk of heart disease, a different strategy is called for. To restore your body's responsiveness to insulin, which has nothing to do with how strong your muscles are or what your heart's stroke volume is, you don't need to build muscles. You just need to use the muscles you have, particularly the slow-twitch muscles that contain all those mitochondria. To do that all you need to do is walk.

BUILDING VERSUS ACTIVATING MUSCLES

One of the reasons we find exercise difficult is that we think we have to be *building* something—strength, endurance, whatever. Sure, if you push yourself, you can increase your strength and endurance. But to reverse insulin resistance, lose weight, and prevent diabetes, you don't need to build muscles, you just need to activate them.

As you exercise, your muscles react to insulin in an interesting way. Nothing happens for several minutes, and then suddenly your muscles start responding. It's like someone flipped a switch. Scientists have actually observed this phenomenon in action using powerful video microscopes to visualize the movements of glucose transporters within cells. At first, the transporters do nothing, and then they suddenly wake up, swarm to the cell surface, and start pulling in glucose from the bloodstream.

The all-or-nothing behavior of insulin sensitivity explains how your body responds to exercise. If you go for a walk, for example, it takes a certain amount of walking to turn on that switch and get your muscles to start responding, but once they do, they respond fully. If you walk more, responsiveness increases a little but not as much as that initial surge. That's why, when it comes to eliminating insulin resistance, you get almost as much benefit by walking a couple of miles (3.2 km) as you do by walking farther.

Of course, you can't just stroll along like you're window-shopping. To activate your insulin switch, you need to walk about as fast as you would if you had an appointment to keep. When you have to be somewhere at a particular time, you make a subconscious calculation: you give yourself enough time to avoid having to run, but you don't tarry, either. Walking at a brisk but comfortable pace puts your slow-twitch muscles to their full use. You turn on your metabolic switch, and you don't get tired because your mitochondria instantly restore the energy you use.

Once you turn on that switch, your muscles remain sensitive to insulin for 24 to 48 hours. Here's the catch: it doesn't matter if you run a marathon or walk a couple of miles, after 48 hours, your muscles lose their responsiveness. If you only exercise on weekends, you spend at least half of the following week in a state of insulin resistance. That's why the U.S. surgeon general recommends walking 30 minutes "most days of the week." That's about 10 miles (16 km) a week.

A few years ago, I saw a photograph in the *Seattle Times* taken in 1915 of a dozen or so businessmen standing in their office. They wore suits—they weren't doing physical work. What caught my eye was that none were overweight. I wondered, what did they do that was different from us to keep from gaining weight? They ate plenty of bread and potatoes; evidence suggests that the average caloric intake then was actually higher than it is now, and they didn't exercise in gyms. The only difference is that most people who worked in down-town Seattle in those days had to walk a couple of miles (3.2 km) to get to work. They were flipping their muscle switches twice a day. (This was when I gave up my downtown parking space and started walking to work.)

Research shows that going from getting no exercise to being a regular walker exceeds the health benefits of going from being a walker to being a runner. Of course, the flip side of exercise being good for you is that being a couch potato is bad for you. Research shows that a sedentary lifestyle is a potent risk factor for obesity, diabetes, polycystic ovary syndrome (PCOS), and heart disease.

Our Fixation on Endurance Exercise

When you think of getting in shape, perhaps the first thing that comes to mind is running. To build endurance, you have to huff and puff and continue huffing and puffing for longer than you would like—maybe 20 or 30 minutes, three or four times a week. This is painful. It requires motivation and discipline. It's especially hard if you're overweight or older than fifty. Few people continue running faithfully into their fifties.

So why has endurance training become synonymous with exercise? Running has the reputation of being good for the heart because how fast and far you can run depends on how much blood your heart can pump with each beat at maximal exertion—stroke volume. Endurance training increases stroke volume. In that sense, it's good for your heart, but here's where the confusion comes in.

The most common kind of heart disease is coronary artery disease—narrowing and blocking of the arteries that supply blood to the heart. When you exercise, your heart muscle needs more blood. If the arteries are narrowed or blocked, it may not get enough blood, which can cause chest pain with exertion, or angina. For years, angina patients were advised to avoid exercise for fear of triggering a heart attack. However, in the 1960s, doctors discovered that endurance training can open up detour channels around coronary artery blockages, improve blood supply to the heart, and reduce angina. The same lack of blood flow to the heart that causes angina also triggers the heart muscle to release growth factors that stimulate the development of new channels. That's how endurance exercise got the reputation of being good for your heart.

However, unless your coronary arteries are narrowed or blocked, your heart already gets plenty of blood when you exercise. You don't need new channels. You need to prevent the buildup of cholesterol and keep your arteries from clogging up in the first place. Indeed, exercise helps prevent cholesterol buildup in your arteries, but not by increasing stroke volume. It works by improving insulin responsiveness, which lowers cholesterol and blood pressure and prevents diabetes. You don't need to be a runner to do that. All you need to do is flip that insulin switch in your muscles, and you can do that by walking. If you don't already have narrow coronary arteries, the only benefit to your heart of all that huffing and puffing is that it increases the amount of blood your heart can pump at maximal exertion.

Actually, walking for exercise also increases your endurance, although not as much as running does. But ask yourself, why do you need super endurance? Unless you're intent on winning foot races, running for exercise doesn't do much more good than walking.

Benefits of Resistance Training

The best way to strengthen muscles is to strain them against resistance. Weight lifting is an example. Resistance exercise uses fast-twitch muscles, which contain less mitochondria than slow-twitch ones. Exercising them doesn't increase insulin sensitivity as much as exercising your slow-twitch muscles does. However, it increases it a little. Studies show that adding resistance exercise to a walking program provides a modest increase in insulin responsiveness.

As you age, your muscles tend to shrink, a process that accelerates in your forties. Muscle-strengthening exercise prevents the loss of muscle mass that occurs with aging. Resistance exercise also toughens muscle attachments and helps prevent overuse injuries from other activities. Having good muscle strength makes the activities of daily living easier, which helps keep you active.

If you're worried that muscle-strengthening exercise will make you look bulky, relax. It's easy for young men to increase their muscle mass because they produce a lot of testosterone, a hormone that promotes muscle growth. However, if you're female or a male older than forty, you don't have enough testosterone in your system to promote an unusually large increase in the size of your muscles. Muscle-strengthening exercise will restore a youthful shape to your muscles—"definition"—but won't make you appear muscle-bound.

A typical strength-building routine is to do two groups of ten repetitions against resistance—such as lifting weights—with the last repetition being against maximal resistance. You can determine maximal resistance by experimentation. Increase the weight you're lifting until you are unable to lift it ten times in a row, and then use the next lowest weight for your repetitions. During resistance training, it's okay to take a breather between sets. Remember, this isn't endurance training; you're not trying to increase your heart's stroke volume.

One good thing about strength training is you don't have to spend much time doing it. A good routine would be to strengthen your upper body muscles with a couple of 30-minute sessions a week and then walk to keep your leg muscles in shape. What about leg-strengthening exercises? The best thing about being overweight is that you have great leg muscles. They're plenty strong already. All you need to do is get those puppies moving by walking, and they'll have a major effect on your metabolism.

DEFEAT PRE-EXERCISE LETHARGY

The three most common problems psychiatrists see these days are depression, anxiety, and inability to stay focused on mental tasks, or attention deficit disorder. Exercise improves all three. It raises the levels of serotonin and other hormones in your nervous system that counteract depression. Studies show that a regular walking program is as good as antidepressant medication for treating mild depression. Exercise is also as effective as tranquilizers for relieving mild anxiety, without the side effects and threats of addiction that tranquilizers pose. Exercise also improves focus, which helps people with attention deficit disorder. Further, it increases production of endorphins, your body's own painkillers, imparting a feeling of calm and well-being that continues for hours after exercise.

Antidepressant, tranquilizer, mental performance enhancer, pain reliever—if exercise were a drug, you couldn't keep people away from it. So why don't we do more of it?

Here's the plain truth: as we age, we develop a natural aversion to exercise. When we're kids, we love to run, jump, and climb trees. We have a hard time sitting still. As we get older, we still enjoy physical activity, but it's less spontaneous—instead of free play, we participate in organized fitness programs and sports. Eventually, we lose the drive to exercise altogether. We'll do it if there's a reason, but we have to force ourselves. We like the *idea* of exercise. It's just that when it comes time to *do* it, we get hit with a dose of lethargy.

If exercise is so good for us, then why does Mother Nature take away our drive to do it as we age, which is when we need it the most? Wouldn't we be better off if we still loved to run, jump, and climb trees for the fun of it? Well, maybe not. In prehistoric times, unless you had to hunt for food, you were better off hunkered down in your cave. Venturing outside wasted energy and exposed you to predators wanting to eat you. If you're comfortable where you are and have no desire to get up and exert yourself, your prehistoric ancestors would understand.

But our cave-dwelling relatives couldn't sit in their caves for long. Sooner or later, they had to get out and compete with the rest of the animal kingdom for food. Sluggishness no longer served them well. Once they emerged from their caves, they needed energy, strength, and a positive attitude to hunt game and gather vegetation.

That's when their hormones kicked in. Once they got out of their caves and started moving, their attitudes changed. Their adrenaline levels surged, strengthening their muscles and quickening their reflexes. Their serotonin levels rose, sharpening their focus and energizing them mentally. Endorphins took away their aches and pains. They were ready for action.

So don't be put off by your own ambivalent attitude toward exercise. We know it makes us feel better, but when it comes time to do it, we seem to have better things to do. This is a normal reaction, and we justify it with weak excuses like not having enough time. I hear that excuse virtually every working day of my life, but I doubt it's the problem. Look around at your local gym. You'll see plenty of people in their twenties and thirties, but not so many in their forties and fifties. The younger ones are starting new jobs and raising kids. Why would they have more time on their hands than folks in their fifties who are established in their jobs and whose kids are out of the house? They don't. The real reason is that exercise expends energy, and, like the caveman hunkered in his cave, your natural instinct is to conserve energy.

There are two ways to deal with this aversion to physical exertion. You can call on your discipline to overcome this lassitude and just *do* it. But most of us don't have that much discipline. The other way is to make exercise easier. Happily, the easiest exercise—walking— is as effective at eliminating insulin resistance as the hardest kinds. The trick is to take that first step. Like a caveman on the hunt, once you start walking, your hormones will kick in and your attitude will change.

6

UNDERSTAND YOUR GLYCEMIC LOAD

I n 1862, an Englishman named William Banting published a pamphlet describing how he succeeded in losing weight by eating freely of meat and vegetables but avoiding bread, potatoes, and rice. The pamphlet became popular in Europe and America, and for years his name was used as a verb. If you were cutting carbohydrates you were said to be "banting." It was generally accepted by the medical profession that obesity was caused by eating starchy and sugary foods and the best way to lose weight was to avoid refined carbohydrates. Then in the 1970s, government agencies and medical organizations started recommending that people reduce their consumption of fat and cholesterol, advice that triggered an epidemic of obesity and diabetes.

It took a savvy New York cardiologist to get people to return to what had worked in the past. In 1992, Robert C. Atkins, M.D., published *Dr. Atkins' New Diet Revolution*. Atkins knew that dietary fat and cholesterol are not what cause heart disease, and the best way to lose weight is to follow the time-honored advice to avoid carbohydrates. He advised his patients to forget about counting calories and instead eat all the eggs, meat, and dairy products they wanted but eliminate all carbohydrates except leafy green vegetables.

Initially, Atkins was criticized by the medical profession for recommending what was deemed a reckless way to eat. Most doctors were convinced that eating so much fat and cholesterol would raise blood cholesterol levels and increase the risk of heart disease. Nevertheless, his diet worked. Dieters discovered that they really could eat as much as they wanted and still lose weight, as long as they avoided carbohydrates. To the medical profession's dismay, increasing numbers of people ignored warnings about fat and cholesterol and went on the Atkins diet. It turned out that folks who follwed Atkins' advice ended up being healthier than ever. The balance between good cholesterol and bad cholesterol, the most accurate predictor of artery problems, actually improved. Blood sugar levels went down, and there was no suggestion of an increase of heart disease.

In 2002, researchers published the results of two large research trials that put the Atkins diet to the test. In each study, they instructed one group of patients to avoid carbohydrates and eat as much meat, eggs, and dairy products as they wanted, and not restrict calories. They instructed another group to reduce dietary fat and cholesterol and restrict calories. These studies confirmed what Atkins said all along: dietary fat and cholesterol do not cause high blood cholesterol or heart problems. Most remarkably, the subjects who eliminated carbohydrates lost weight *without trying to reduce calories.* Even though they ate all they wanted, they lost more weight than the subjects on low-fat diets who tried to cut calories. Reducing carbohydrates lowered their insulin levels, which allowed nutrients to reach the brain and satisfy their hunger, rather than being pushed into their fat cells by insulin.

THE DOWNSIDE OF RADICAL, LOW-CARB DIETS

The Atkins diet was wildly popular for several years, but eventually fell from grace. The problem was *food cravings*. Atkins advised eliminating virtually all carbohydrates—not just starch and sugar but also fruit and vegetables. The only carbohydrates the diet allowed were limited amounts of leafy green vegetables. To put this in perspective, the average American consumes 250 to 300 grams of carbohydrates per day. Atkins recommended eating fewer than 20 grams per day. People who start the Atkins diet are typically pleased at first because they can eat their fill of rich food, but after a week or two, they usually start longing for the missing foods and slip back to their old ways.

The problem with the Atkins and other radical, low-carb diets is that they defy deep biological urges. Fruits and vegetables contain vitamins, minerals, and fiber that are essential to good health. If you don't have enough of these in your diet, you eventually develop serious health problems. However, your body doesn't let that happen. Natural cravings protect you from vitamin and mineral deficiencies long before they actually occur, which is why Atkins dieters started longing for their missing foods, even though they weren't having harmful deficiencies. There's even a biological basis for craving sweets. To our prehistoric ancestors, the taste of sugar indicated that a plant contained calories and was safe to eat.

Medical science has come a long way toward understanding the effects of different foods on insulin production since Atkins published his book. It turns out that you don't have to go on a strict, low-carb diet to lose weight and reverse insulin resistance. There is a way to enjoy tasty foods—including fruit, vegetables, and sweets—while minimizing your insulin levels and losing weight, and it's a much more natural way to eat. It's all about reducing your *glycemic load*.

UNDERSTANDING GLYCEMIC LOAD

To Atkins and the scientists of his time, a carb was a carb. It made no difference whether you consumed carbohydrates in fruits and vegetables or in potatoes and candy. All that mattered was how much glucose the carbohydrates released into your bloodstream. If you wanted to reduce your insulin levels, you had to avoid all carbohydrates.

Several years after the Atkins diet became popular, scientists developed the means to measure the amount of insulin the body produces in response to different foods. They discovered that when it comes to raising insulin levels, not all carbs are the same. Some cause the body to produce more insulin than others, even if they release the same amount of glucose into the bloodstream. For example, 50 grams of carbohydrates in bread raise blood glucose and insulin levels higher than 50 grams of carbohydrates in broccoli, even though they ultimately release the same amount of glucose into the bloodstream.

The reason for these differences is that some carbs are broken down and absorbed into your bloodstream faster than others. The speed of absorption is influenced by such things as chemical structure, cellulose barriers, fiber content, particle size, liquidity, and acidity. The only sure way to predict how much a particular food will raise blood glucose and insulin levels is to have human subjects eat the food and measure glucose and insulin levels afterward. Scientists have now done this on hundreds of foods and produced a ranking system for the effects that different foods have on blood glucose and insulin levels. It's called the *glycemic index.*

The glycemic index compares the effects of different carbohydrates to a standard—usually white bread. White bread is assigned a value of 100, and the comparison foods are given a number that represents their effect on blood glucose levels compared with that of white bread. For example, peas have a glycemic index of 73, which means 50 grams of carbohydrates that enter your bloodstream after consuming peas raises blood glucose 73 percent as much as 50 grams of carbohydrates entering your blood after consuming white bread.

The Critical Difference Between Glycemic Index and Glycemic Load

The glycemic index provided useful insights into the effects of various foods on blood glucose levels. However, the scientists who developed it never meant for it to be used as a dietary guide. They were trying to prove a point—that different foods raise blood glucose and insulin levels more than others do, even though they release the same amount of glucose into the bloodstream. To accomplish this, they needed to give subjects the same amount of digestible carbohydrates in each food they tested so they arbitrarily chose 50 grams of carbohydrates as the standard.

The problem is that the amounts of food subjects had to eat to get to 50 grams of carbohydrates bears no relationship to the way people typically eat. To absorb 50 grams of carbohydrates in carrots, a person has to eat seven full-size carrots—a lot more than most folks eat in one sitting.

Thus, a few years later, scientists developed a more useful measurement called the *glycemic load.* Unlike the glycemic index, the glycemic load reflects the effects on blood glucose and insulin levels of amounts of food people typically eat. For example, the glycemic load of a carrot reflects the effects of eating a single carrot—an amount a person would actually eat.

The difference between the glycemic index and glycemic load might seem like technical nitpicking. A lot of doctors brushed over what seemed like a minor adjustment. However, the glycemic load measurements provide astonishing insights into why we develop obesity, diabetes, and polycystic ovary syndrome (PCOS). These problems correlate more strongly with the glycemic load than with any other dietary measurement, including carbohydrate content, glycemic index, or fat content, and reducing glycemic load has proven effective for reversing all of these conditions.

THE CULPRITS REVEALED

When you look at food through the lens of glycemic load, the cause of Americans' dietary problems becomes much clearer. All but a fraction of the glycemic load of the typical American diet come from two substances: starch, the main sources of which are flour products, potatoes, and rice, and sugar-containing beverages, mainly soda and fruit juices.

Although sodas are a big problem for kids, most grown-ups the least bit concerned about their weight have given up drinking them or have switched to diet pop. Indeed, the main problem for adults is starch—flour products, potatoes, and rice. In a study of the diets of 78,000 American women, researchers found that the total glycemic load of the starches these women ate was more than twenty times that of any other food, including sugar and candy.

The following table lists the glycemic loads of fifty-nine common foods (a more complete list is provided in the appendix). The serving sizes of these foods are estimates of the amounts people typically eat at one sitting. For example, a typical serving of bread would be two slices, as in a sandwich. Note that the glycemic loads in this book are expressed as percentages of the blood-glucose-raising effect of a single ¼-inch (6 mm) thick slice of white bread. For example, the glycemic load of an apple is 78, which means an average size apple raises blood glucose 78 percent as much as a ¼-inch (6 mm) thick slice of white bread would. To convert the glycemic load values on other listings, such as the International Table of Glycemic Indexes and Loads, to the percentages I use throughout this book, multiply those values by 10. The sizes I have listed reflect typical American servings, which are sometimes different from international listings.

GLYCEMIC LOADS OF COMMON FOODS
(Compared to a 1-oz [28 g] slice of white bread)

Food item	Description	Typical serving	Glycemic load (% of white bread)
Pancake	1 (5-inch [12.5 cm]) diameter	2½ oz (70 g)	346
Bagel	1 medium size	3⅓ oz (90 g)	340
Orange soda	12-oz (355 ml) can	12 oz (355 ml)	314
Macaroni	2 cups (280 g)	10 oz (280 g)	301
White rice	1 cup (182 g)	6½ oz (182 g)	283
Spaghetti	2 cups (280 g)	10 oz (280 g)	276
White bread	2 slices, ⅜-inch (1 cm) thick	2¾ oz (78 g)	260
Baked potato	1 medium	5 oz (140 g)	246
Whole-wheat bread	2 slices, ⅜-inch (1 cm) thick	2¾ oz (78 g)	234
Raisin Bran	1 cup (59 g)	2 oz (56 g)	227
Brown rice	1 cup (182 g)	6½ oz (182 g)	222
French fries	large serving (McDonald's)	5.9 oz (168 g)	219
Coca-Cola	12-oz (355 ml) can	12 oz (355 ml)	218
Hamburger bun	Top and bottom, 5-inch (12.5 cm) diameter	2½ oz (70 g)	213
English muffin	1 medium	2 oz (56 g)	208
Doughnut	1 medium	2 oz (56 g)	205
Corn Flakes	1 cup (28 g)	1 oz (28 g)	199
Corn on the cob	1 ear	5⅓ oz (150 g)	171
Blueberry muffin	2½-inch (6.4 cm) diameter	2 oz (56 g)	169
Instant oatmeal (cooked)	1 cup (227 g)	8 oz (227 g)	154

(continued)

Food item	Description	Typical serving	Glycemic load (% of white bread)
Chocolate cake	1 (4 × 4 × 1-inch [10 × 10 × 2.5 cm]) slice	3 oz (84 g)	154
Grape-Nuts	1 cup (116 g)	4 oz (116 g)	142
Cheerios	1 cup (28 g)	1 oz (28 g)	142
Special K	1 cup (31 g)	1 oz (28 g)	133
Cookie	1 medium	1 oz (28 g)	114
White bread (standard)	1 slice, ¼-inch (0.6 cm) thick	1 oz (28 g)	100
Tortilla (corn)	1 medium	1¼ oz (35 g)	85
Banana	1 medium	3¼ oz (93 g)	85
All-Bran	½ cup (31 g)	1 oz (28 g)	85
Tortilla (wheat)	1 medium	1¾ oz (49 g)	80
Apple	1 medium	5½ oz (154 g)	78
Grapefruit juice (unsweetened)	6-oz (175 ml) glass	6 oz (175 ml)	75
Orange	1 medium	6 oz (168 g)	71
Pinto beans	½ cup (84 g)	3 oz (84 g)	57
Pear	1 medium	6 oz (168 g)	57
Pineapple	1 slice (¾-inch thick × 3½-inch wide [2 × 9 cm])	3 oz (84 g)	50
Peach	1 medium	4 oz (112 g)	47
Grapes	1 cup (40 grapes [70 g])	2½ oz (70 g)	47
Kidney beans	½ cup (84 g)	3 oz (84 g)	40
Grapefruit	1 half	4½ oz (126 g)	32
Table sugar	1 rounded teaspoon (4 g)	⅙ oz (4 g)	28
Milk (whole)	8-oz (235 ml) glass	8 oz (235 ml)	27

(continued)

Food item	Description	Typical serving	Glycemic load (% of white bread)
Peas	¼ cup (38 g)	1½ oz (42 g)	16
Tomato	1 medium	5 oz (140 g)	15
Strawberries	1 cup (145 g)	5½ oz (154 g)	13
Carrot (raw)	1 medium (7½ inches [19 cm])	3 oz (84 g)	11
Peanuts	¼ cup (37 g)	1¼ oz (35 g)	7
Spinach	1 cup (70 g)	2½ oz (70 g)	0
Pork	Two 5-oz (140 g) chops	10 oz (280 g)	0
Margarine	1½ teaspoons (7 g)	¼ oz (7 g)	0
Lettuce	1 cup (70 g)	2½ oz (70 g)	0
Fish	8-oz (227 g) fillet	8 oz (227 g)	0
Eggs	1	1½ oz (42 g)	0
Cucumber	1 cup (168 g)	6 oz (168 g)	0
Chicken	1 breast	10 oz (280 g)	0
Cheese	2 × 2 × 1-inch (5 × 5 × 2.5 cm) slice	2 oz (56 g)	0
Butter	1½ teaspoons (7 g)	¼ oz (7 g)	0
Broccoli	½ cup (35 g)	1½ oz (42 g)	0
Beef	10-oz (280 g) steak	10 oz (280 g)	0

Source: Rob Thompson, M.D. The glycemic loads in this book are expressed as percentages of the blood-glucose-raising effect of a single ¼-inch (6 mm) thick slice of white bread and reflect typical American servings, which sometimes differ from international listings. See page 43 for more information. Note: Per serving gram amounts may vary depending on source and food preparation methods.

LIMIT FLOUR PRODUCTS, POTATOES, AND RICE

You can see that the glycemic loads of bread, potatoes, and rice are several times higher than fruits and vegetables. The Atkins diet forbids fruits—they're carbohydrates, too—but notice that you would have to eat six pears in one sitting to give you the glycemic load you get from one bagel. You would have to consume five peaches to equal the glycemic load of a sandwich. You can see that when it comes to reducing glycemic load, it makes little sense to worry about fruit and vegetables if you're still eating flour products, potatoes, and rice. It turns out that most of us can reduce our glycemic load to a fraction of what it was by just avoiding these three foods. This is why the latest U.S. Food and Drug Administration's *Dietary Guidelines for Americans* recommends focusing on reducing refined carbohydrates and not worrying about dietary fat and cholesterol.

Look again at the foods with glycemic loads of 100 or more. Do you see a pattern? They're mostly all grain products. An exception is potatoes, which are similar to grains in that their job in nature is to supply energy for plants to sprout. Now look at the foods with glycemic loads less than 100: almost everything *but* grain products. If a caveman could see the list, he would recognize many of the foods with glycemic loads less than 100. Humans have been eating meat, fish, eggs, nuts, fruit, and vegetables for millions of years. He wouldn't recognize most of the foods with glycemic loads higher than 100. They're mainly grain products, and grains weren't part of the prehistoric diet.

Notice that most of the foods with glycemic loads of less than 100 are perishable. They're not the kind of foods you can wrap in cellophane and store on a shelf for weeks as you can with most foods at the top of the list. These come in the form in which they are harvested— they're not processed. Most of the foods with glycemic loads higher than 100 have been separated from their natural components, pulverized, mixed with other ingredients, and cooked before you eat them.

Starch, a Most Peculiar Food

The word *starch* comes from the Old English word *sterchen*—to stiffen. It's the same substance used for stiffening shirt collars (which, ironically, is what it does to your arteries). One of the weirdest things about starch is that it's 98 percent tasteless. About 2 percent of it turns into glucose in your mouth, which you can taste, but otherwise, your taste buds don't respond to it. If you want to prove that to yourself, try eating a spoonful of flour. It's nearly tasteless. Most of the flavor in the starches you eat comes from added ingredients, such as fat, sugar, salt, and spices.

Because the glucose molecules in starch are bound to one another, they can't interact with the taste buds in your mouth. Your saliva contains small amounts of the enzyme *amylase*, which frees up about 2 percent of the glucose, which provides a little taste. However, the remaining 98 percent is tasteless.

So what's wrong with not tasting the food you eat? Scientists have discovered that the less taste bud stimulation you get from a food, the more you tend to overeat it. In one experiment, researchers infused food directly into subjects' stomachs through tubes. They found that food that bypasses the taste buds doesn't reduce hunger as much as food that interacts with them.

Ironically, as tasteless as starch is, as soon as it reaches your intestine, it turns into sugar. Imagine eating a pile of sugar the size of a couple slices of bread, a potato, or a serving of rice. Essentially, that's what you are doing when you eat those foods. As one researcher put it, you can put a teaspoon of sugar on a bowl of Wheaties or a teaspoon of Wheaties on a bowl of sugar. In the end, it's all the same. Starch raises your blood sugar and insulin levels as much as similar amounts of pure sugar.

Another peculiar characteristic of starch is that it's completely absorbed in the first foot or two (30 to 60 cm) of your intestine. Whereas most other foods traverse the full 26 feet (8 m) of your intestinal tract as they are being taken up by your bloodstream, starch never gets to the last part of your intestine. Normally, when partially digested food reaches this part of your intestine, cells lining the intestinal wall send hormones to the appetite-control centers in your brain, telling them that you've eaten enough. Scientists call this appetite-control mechanism the "intestinal brake" because it puts the brakes on eating when your intestines have all the food they can handle. Starch bypasses that regulating system altogether.

Wheat, our main source of starch, also contains *gluten,* a protein that can trigger a harmful immune response in susceptible individuals. Although uncommon, gluten intolerance can cause a host of medical problems, including chronic indigestion, malnutrition, and anemia. Because gluten intolerance is difficult to diagnose, many people who have it don't know it. Some experts think gluten might cause subtler problems, such as intermittent diarrhea, tiredness, and poor concentration, in more people than previously suspected.

Unlike most of the food we eat, starch contains no vital nutrients. No creature has ever suffered poor health due to lack of starch. Our prehistoric ancestors existed for millions of years without it. Whatever genetic adaptations might be needed to accommodate our dependence on starch have not had time to occur. Indeed, when humans started relying on starch rather than animal fat and protein for sustenance, they became shorter in stature, less muscular, and prone to what are known as diseases of civilization, including obesity, diabetes, and PCOS.

The High Price of Cheap Food

The reason modern humans eat so much starch is that it provides more calories with less investment of land, labor, and capital than any other type of food. People in most parts of the world have come to depend on starchy staples, such as wheat, potatoes, and rice, for their very survival.

An economist looking at the list of glycemic loads might notice that although the foods with glycemic loads greater than 100 are not necessarily cheap, they're made of cheap ingredients. For example, the ingredients in breakfast cereals—grain, sugar, salt, flavoring—comprise a small fraction of the amount of money you end up paying for them. In other words, there's potential profit in getting you to eat them.

Sugar-Containing Beverages

You can see there's one other kind of food (if you call it a food) that's high on the glycemic load list—soda. Regular consumption of non-diet sodas is strongly associated with obesity and diabetes. One study found that women who consumed one or more non-diet sodas daily for ten years doubled their risk of diabetes and gained an average of 18 pounds (8 kg) more than women who didn't drink soda.

Prehistoric humans had nothing in their diet resembling sugar-containing beverages. Like every other creature on earth, their only beverage was water. Even until recently, people drank mainly coffee, tea, milk, or water. Soda and fruit juice were occasional treats. In the last fifty years, thanks to cheap ingredients and modern technology, soda and fruit juice consumption has increased dramatically, along with epidemics of obesity and diabetes. Sugar-containing beverages comprise a significant portion of the caloric intake of children and teenagers and are strongly associated with childhood obesity and diabetes.

The main problem with sugar-containing beverages is that, like starch, you taste only a fraction of the sugar in them. This is because your digestive system handles liquids differently than solids. When you chew food, you roll it against your tongue, which allows the ingredients to stimulate your taste buds. However, most of the sugar in liquids flies over your tongue and down your throat without coming into contact with your taste buds. We also add sour ingredients, such as lemon or lime juice, to beverages, which hides the sweetness of the sugar in them. As a result, we end up consuming phenomenal amounts of sugar. For example, a 12-ounce (355 ml) can of cola contains 10 teaspoons (40 g) of sugar. Imagine trying to eat that much sugar right out of the sugar bowl.

What about diet sodas? They have little effect on blood sugar or insulin levels. Although some scientists have expressed concern about possible harmful effects of the artificial sweeteners used in them, millions of people drink diet sodas, and so far they haven't been proven to cause any health problems.

Sodas aren't the only beverage that will raise your blood sugar and insulin levels. Fruit juices are also high on the glycemic load list, even without added sugar. When you squeeze the sugar out of a half dozen oranges or apples and put it in a glass, you end up with a sugar-sweetened, high-glycemic-load beverage. Orange juice raises blood sugar so quickly and reliably that diabetics often use it to raise their blood sugar when they've taken too much insulin.

Ounce for ounce, orange and apple juices contain almost as much sugar as Coca-Cola. It may be natural sugar—it wasn't added by manufacturers—but it's sugar nonetheless. As far as science knows, there's no difference between natural sugar and sugar that comes in a box. Like sodas, daily consumption of fruit juices is linked to obesity and diabetes, not to mention tooth decay.

Liquids Don't Satisfy Hunger

Sugar-containing beverages provide calories but don't reduce the amount of food you eat. In one study, researchers fed subjects 300 calories in jelly beans every day for six weeks and compared them to subjects fed 300 calories a day in beverages. The subjects who ate the jelly beans reduced their daily consumption of calories from other foods by approximately the same amount of calories in the jelly beans. However, the subjects who consumed added calories in beverage form did not reduce their consumption of other foods at all.

Your digestive system has to change solids into liquids before they can be absorbed into your bloodstream. Sugar-containing beverages are ready for absorption as soon as they reach your intestine. They skip the whole digestive process and pass directly into your bloodstream.

Sugar-containing beverages and starch are alike in several ways. Both are unnatural foods. Prehistoric humans had nothing in their diet resembling them. Both contain large amounts of sugar you can't taste. Both are digested faster than other kinds of food. Unlike other kinds of food, both short-circuit into your bloodstream in the first foot or two (30 to 60 cm) of your intestine. Both cause your body to produce unnaturally large amounts of insulin, and both are strongly associated with obesity and diabetes.

HOW SUGAR CAN WORK FOR YOU

From the time we were kids, our parents lectured us about the evils of sugar (sucrose). But it wasn't because they were afraid we would get fat or diabetic. It was because sugar causes tooth decay. Sugar is easy to digest, not only by you but also by the bacteria in your mouth. When they metabolize sugar, they produce lactic acid as a by-product. Constant exposure to acid dissolves the enamel coating on our teeth, which can create small holes or cavities.

Consequently, the pattern in which you consume sugar is important. An occasional sugary snack isn't hard on your teeth—it's constant exposure that does the damage. Your saliva is alkaline; it neutralizes the acids that bacteria produce when you eat sugar. After a few hours, your enamel recovers. However, if your teeth are constantly exposed to acid, your enamel doesn't have a chance to repair itself, which is when you develop tooth decay.

Actually, if sugar is not mixed with starch, consumed in a beverage, or constantly in your mouth, it's not the evil substance it's often made out to be. Indeed, it can actually be a helpful part of your diet. Here's how.

The tongue is designed to detect small concentrations of sugar; large amounts can be overwhelming. It doesn't take much to satisfy a craving for something sweet. However, it's another story when sugar is mixed with starch—as in cookies, cakes, or pastries. Starch blunts the sweetness of added sugar and keeps it from interacting with your taste buds. You can't taste much sugar, so you end up needing higher concentrations to satisfy your urge for something sweet. You end up eating more sugar, and that's in addition to the glucose that starch releases when it arrives in your intestinal tract.

However, when sugar is not diluted by flour or water, we really don't need much of it to satisfy our urge for something sweet. Chocolate, for example, contains sugar, but because the sugar isn't diluted by starch or water, you taste more of it. A 2 × 2-inch (5 × 5 cm) square of Ghirardelli's dark chocolate contains approximately ½ teaspoon (2 g) of sugar. A couple of squares should be enough to satisfy a sweet tooth—and the glycemic load is less than 33 percent of that of a slice of white bread. The glycemic load of a teaspoon (4 g) of sugar is only 28—one-fourth that of a slice of bread.

You can make a serving of berries taste ripe by sprinkling ½ teaspoon (2 g) of sugar on them. The glycemic load of the added sugar is about 14—one-seventh that of a slice of bread. In both cases, you enjoy sugar's sweetness without raising your glycemic load enough to worry about it. If you use sugar as a way to satisfy the urge for something sweet—not to quench your thirst or satisfy your hunger—you only need a little of it.

Here's how sweets can actually work for you. The tiny bit of glucose that bread, potatoes, or rice release in your mouth provides enough sweetness that many of us have a hard time resisting. Sugar is the cure for that craving. If, instead of eating a pile of potatoes or rice in order to taste the 2 percent that turns into glucose in your mouth, you eat something really sweet—a couple of squares of chocolate or a few jelly beans—you lose your desire for whatever sweetness you might get from starch. This is where dessert comes in. A couple of squares of dark chocolate can satisfy your urge for something sweet and mark the end of a meal.

STARCH: WHY CAN'T WE GIVE IT UP?

Because you don't taste 98 percent of the starch you eat, it contributes little to the flavor of your diet. When you replace it with other foods, you actually increase the amount of flavor in your diet. You end up eating richer, tastier foods. So what is it about starch that makes it difficult for some folks to give up?

Our attraction to starch comes from the way we were fed when we were young. Food preferences are formed in early childhood. A baby's first solid foods need to be easily digestible, and the easiest solid foods to digest are starches. Bread, potatoes, and rice were among the first solid foods our parents fed us when we were being weaned from milk. It's not surprising that we never lose our taste for them.

Here's the good news: you don't have to abstain from any food, including starches, to lower your glycemic load. If you understand the glycemic load and implement the following advice, here's what will happen:

- You will add flavor to your diet.
- You will add vital nutrients to your diet.
- You will continue to enjoy sweets.
- You will eat enough starch to keep you from craving it.
- Your body's demands for insulin will plummet.
- You will lose weight.
- Your belly will shrink.
- You will reverse the main cause of diabetes, gout, PCOS in women, and erectile dysfunction and low testosterone in men.
- No one will notice that you're eating differently than you were before.

THE MAGIC NUMBER: 500

When you eat a carbohydrate, your blood glucose level starts rising in a few minutes, peaks in a couple of hours, and returns to normal in three or four hours. The glycemic load is an estimate of how high your blood glucose rises. The amount of insulin your beta cells secrete in a day reflects the total of the glycemic loads of the food you eat that day.

The table opposite lists the glycemic loads of foods a hypothetical person might eat in a day. Notice that the total daily glycemic load, 2095, is the sum of the glycemic loads of all the foods consumed that day.

Studies show that the risk of obesity, diabetes, heart disease, and PCOS correlates better with the average daily total of the glycemic loads than with any other dietary measurement, including calories, fat, or total carbohydrates. Success in treating those conditions depends on how successful you are at lowering your glycemic load.

How high can your daily glycemic load go without causing your body to produce harmful amounts of insulin? Studies show that the risk of problems related to insulin excess increases as the average daily glycemic load exceeds 500. Moreover, for overweight individuals, daily glycemic loads less than 500 reliably produce weight loss.

EXAMPLE OF TOTAL DAILY GLYCEMIC LOAD	
Food	**Glycemic load (percent of a slice of bread)**
Breakfast	
Orange juice	68
Bagel	340
Lunch	
Turkey sandwich	260
Potato chips	77
Cola	218
Snack	
Corn chips	97
Doughnut	205
Dinner	
Caesar salad (with croutons)	100
Spaghetti	276
French bread	284
Butter	0
Red wine	0
Dessert	
Cookie	114
Total glycemic load	**2,039**

Source: Rob Thompson, M.D. The glycemic loads in this book are expressed as percentages of the blood-glucose-raising effect of a single ¼-inch (6 mm) thick slice of white bread and reflect typical American servings, which sometimes differ from international listings. See page 43 for more information. Note: Per serving gram amounts may vary depending on source and food preparation methods.

SMALL CHANGES THAT PRODUCE BIG RESULTS

Keeping your daily glycemic load less than 500 is so easy that some days you probably do it unintentionally. To illustrate, the table below compares a typical day's menu for a hypothetical person who's not paying attention to glycemic load with a person eating just as heartily but sticking to foods with lower glycemic loads. Notice how well you can eat yet end up with a total glycemic load that is a fraction of what it would be if you ate a few extra high-glycemic-load culprits. Modest changes in your diet can produce dramatic changes in glycemic load.

LOW GLYCEMIC LOAD VERSUS TYPICAL EATING PATTERN

Low-glycemic-load pattern	Glycemic load (percent of a slice of white bread)	Typical pattern	Glycemic load (percent of a slice of white bread)
Breakfast		**Breakfast**	
Bacon	0	Orange juice	68
Eggs	0	Bagel	340
Coffee	0	Coffee	0
Buttered toast	100	Sugar, 1 tsp (4 g)	28
Sugar, 1 tsp (4 g)	28		
Snack		**Snack**	
Latte	27	Coffee	0
Apple	78	Sugar, 1 tsp (4 g)	28
		Doughnut	205
Lunch		**Lunch**	
Chicken Caesar salad (no croutons)	0	Turkey sandwich	260
Milk	27	Potato chips	77
		Coca-Cola	218
Snack		**Snack**	
Mixed nuts	7	Corn chips	97

(continued)

Low-glycemic-load pattern	Glycemic load (percent of a slice of white bread)	Typical pattern	Glycemic load (percent of a slice of white bread)
Dinner		**Dinner**	
Green salad	0	Caesar salad (with croutons)	100
12-oz (340 g) steak	0	Spaghetti (2 cups [280 g])	276
Mushrooms	0	French bread	284
Asparagus	0	Butter	0
½ of a baked potato	120	Red wine	0
Butter	0	Cookie	114
Sour cream	0		
Red wine	0		
Dark chocolate	68		
Total glycemic load	**455**	**Total glycemic load**	**2,095**

Note: Rob Thompson, M.D. The glycemic loads in this book are expressed as percentages of the blood-glucose-raising effect of a single ¼-inch (6 mm) thick slice of white bread and reflect typical American servings, which sometimes differ from international listings. See page 43 for more information. Note: Per serving gram amounts may vary depending on source and food preparation methods.

Should you cut out starch altogether? It wouldn't hurt you a bit; no one has ever suffered a day's illness for lack of starch. However, the reality is if you try to eliminate any food entirely, it's human nature to start wanting it more. But you can still have a little starch—in the above example, a piece of toast with breakfast and a half potato at dinner—and still keep your total glycemic load less than 500. Eating a modest portion of the culprit foods reminds you that there's nothing special about them and helps avoid food cravings.

The One-Serving Rule

You can count up the glycemic loads of everything you eat if you want, but the beauty of the glycemic load is that you really only need to keep track of three foods—flour products, potatoes, and rice. It's easy to keep your daily glycemic load under 500 if you follow this simple rule: eat no more than one full serving of starch a day. That can be two half-servings or three one-third servings, as long as it adds up to one. If you stick to one serving a day you can pretty much eat anything else you want—fruits, vegetables, meat, eggs, dairy products, nuts, even a couple of pieces of chocolate—and not exceed 500, at least not by much.

Package Labels: The Rule of 13

The U.S. Food and Drug Administration (FDA) has considered requiring packaged food producers to provide glycemic load estimates on the labels of their products, but decided against it for now. The problem is that it's difficult to measure the glycemic load of a food without actually testing it in human volunteers—something food manufacturers aren't prepared to do. However, you can draw useful conclusions about the glycemic loads of foods from the information on package labels. Just remember the unlucky number 13. That's how many grams of carbohydrates are in a slice of white bread. Nothing delivers glucose into your bloodstream faster than white bread, so *if something contains fewer than 13 grams of carbohydrates, its glycemic load cannot be higher than 100*, which is the glycemic load of a slice of white bread.

Fiber is not digested, so it doesn't contribute to glycemic load. When checking the grams of carbohydrates in a food, *subtract the fiber grams*. For example, ⅓ cup (20 g) of bran cereal contains 15 grams of carbohydrates, but 7 grams of that is fiber. That leaves 8 grams of digestible carbohydrates.

GLYCEMIC LOAD TRICKS

Reducing your glycemic load is the least socially cumbersome way to lose weight. You don't have to worry about being invited to someone's home for dinner or eating out with your friends. Who's going to notice if you take only a few bites of potato or pass up the bread plate? You can lead a low-glycemic-load lifestyle without anyone noticing. Here are a few tricks to help you enjoy meals while reducing your glycemic load.

Pizza

Understanding the principle of glycemic load allows you to eat some things you might have thought were off the menu forever. Take pizza, for example. The best part of the pizza, the topping, contains plenty of fat and cholesterol but few carbohydrates. If you're trying to reduce your glycemic load, the only part you need to worry about is the crust.

The breading in one slice of pizza has a glycemic load of approximately 60 percent of that of a slice of bread. However, notice that the outer edge crust of each slice contains at least two-thirds of the breading. If you don't eat that part—if you just eat the topping and the breading that's directly underneath it—you reduce the glycemic load of each slice to approximately 20. You end up leaving a big pile of pizza crust on your plate, but that's okay. It's a small price to keep from flooding your system with glucose. If your friends complain that you got more topping than they did, tell them you'll leave the tip.

Hamburgers

In the past, hamburgers got a bad rap because of their fat and cholesterol content, but remember: you're not worried about that. You just don't want to spike your blood sugar. It turns out that the only part of a hamburger you need to worry about is the bun, which contains approximately 25 grams of carbohydrates (about twice that in a slice of white bread). Notice that the top bun contains about two-thirds of the breading. If you eliminate it, you end up with about 9 grams of carbohydrates (approximately two-thirds of that of a slice of white bread). Using the rule of 13, you figure that the maximal glycemic load is approximately 66 percent of that of a slice of white bread—not bad. Actually, as you will learn in the next chapter, other ingredients in the burger slow the absorption of carbohydrates and lower the glycemic load even more.

You've done your math; now your only challenge is to figure out how to eat your hamburger without a top bun. One way to do it is to just remove the top bun and eat the burger with a knife and fork. Another method is to pick the burger up and eat it like you normally would, but each time you go to take a bite, you tear a piece of the top bun away from the part you're going to bite.

You can also ask the cook to prepare your burger without any bun at all. Restaurants these days are used to this. They'll even wrap it in a piece of lettuce so you can eat it like a regular hamburger. Either way, you'll probably like the burger better without all that tasteless starch getting in the way of the good stuff.

Sandwiches

Sandwiches are a major contributor to the daily glycemic load of many people. Restaurants try to impress us with the size of their sandwiches, but it's usually not the meat, lettuce, and tomatoes that make them big, it's the bread. The slices are often twice the size of a standard 1-ounce (28 g) slice. Two double-size slices add up to a glycemic load of 400. If you're trying to keep your daily glycemic load below 500, you've almost shot your limit for the day.

One solution is to have a wrap, a sandwich made with a tortilla. A small flour tortilla (6 inches [15 cm] in diameter) has a glycemic load of approximately 86. You can also buy low-carb tortillas, which have estimated glycemic loads below 30—virtually insignificant. Just wrap the tortilla around your ingredients, fold one end so the contents don't fall out, and eat it like a hot dog.

Build a "Starch Pile"

What about mixed dishes such as casseroles? The starchy parts of such dishes are usually easy to see and separate from other ingredients with a knife and fork. You can build a pile of starch on one side of your plate as you eat the other ingredients. When you've finished eating everything else, you can take a few bites of the starch. However, you probably won't find it very exciting once your hunger has been satisfied with other food. At the end of your meal, you can look at your starch pile and congratulate yourself on the tasteless carbs you passed up.

Candy

If a sugary treat has an ingredient list, remember the rule of 13. If it contains less than 13 grams of carbohydrates, then it cannot have a glycemic load greater than 100, the glycemic load of a slice of bread. If there's no ingredient list, here's a rule of thumb (or I should say fist) that will keep you from overeating sweets. No matter how sugary or starchy something is, if you eat no more than you can wrap the fingers of one hand around, its glycemic load is unlikely to exceed 100. Consider jelly beans, which are about as sugary as you can get. If you only eat an amount you can wrap the fingers of one hand around—about five pieces—you consume about 10 grams of carbohydrates. Compare that with a baked potato, which delivers 50 grams. Applying the rule of 13, the glycemic load of the jelly beans can't be more than 77 percent of that of a slice of white bread (10 divided by 13).

Actually, the glycemic loads of some popular sweets are surprisingly low. Chocolate-covered nuts? No problem. Nuts have low glycemic loads and covering them in dark chocolate doesn't add much. Don't worry about the calories. Remember, you're just trying to reduce your insulin production.

A word of warning: sugary sweets seem to have an addictive quality for some of us. We're not satisfied with a few bites. If we have any sweets, we end up eating too much. In talking to people about their diets, I find this behavior uncommon. However, if you have a hard time stopping once you've started eating sweets, you may be better off abstaining completely. Individuals with this impulse say that the craving for sweets subsides after a few weeks of avoiding them altogether.

Remember, diet is only half of the story. You need to keep your muscles sensitive to insulin with regular activation of your slow-twitch muscles. If you do what the U.S. surgeon general suggests and walk 30 minutes on most days of the week, and keep your daily glycemic load under 500, you will eliminate insulin resistance, drop your insulin levels, and steadily lose weight. Your blood glucose will fall and your hormones will come back into balance. It's as easy as that.

7 CARB BLOCKERS

As discussed in the previous chapter, carbohydrates that have low glycemic loads release glucose into your bloodstream more slowly than carbs that have high glycemic loads. Take broccoli, for example. There's nothing different about the glucose in it, but broccoli contains substances and structures that slow the digestion of glucose. The fiber in broccoli soaks up glucose, which keeps it from coming into contact with the intestinal lining, where it is absorbed. It turns out that such "carb-blocking" substances not only slow absorption of glucose released by the foods that contain them, but also the glucose released by other carbohydrates consumed with them. The fiber in broccoli slows the absorption of glucose in bread consumed with it.

Structural characteristics, such as the size of food particles and the presence of cellulose compartments, also affect the speed with which food is digested. Food needs to be liquefied before it can pass into your intestines, where it is absorbed into your bloodstream. The ease with which food breaks down into small particles affects how quickly it can proceed.

The glycemic load of carbohydrates, described in the previous chapter—accounts for about two-thirds of their effects on glucose and insulin levels. The remaining one-third depends on other things, including carb-blocking substances from other foods.

STARCH-BLOCKING MEDICATION

In the 1980s, the pharmaceutical company Bayer began marketing a medication that slows the digestion of starch. Named acarbose, it was used for treating diabetes. Acarbose works by blocking *amylase*, the intestinal enzyme that breaks down starch into glucose.

Acarbose is a natural substance produced by bacteria in soil. It's simply a small piece of starch modified in such a way that when amylase tries to break it down, it ties up the amylase and takes it out of action. Enough amylase remains to digest whatever starch is consumed, but the process takes longer. Essentially, acarbose makes high-glycemic-load foods behave more like low-glycemic-load foods. By slowing the absorption of starch, it reduces after-meal blood glucose and insulin levels.

In addition to helping treat diabetes, acarbose promotes weight loss and reduces blood pressure. It also restores normal ovulation in women with polycystic ovary syndrome (PCOS). And several studies show that acarbose helps prevents heart attacks in patients with mild diabetes.

The problem is that acarbose entered the market before doctors knew about the importance of the glycemic load of carbohydrates. When studies showed that acarbose did not prevent starch absorption—it only slowed it—its popularity declined. Most doctors saw little point in slowing the digestion of starch when it all eventually got digested anyway.

Unfortunately, acarbose's patent expired before scientists discovered how effective it is at treating the complications of insulin resistance. When a drug's patent expires, the company that introduced it to the market no longer has a monopoly on it. Other companies can then compete, which lowers the price significantly. Profit margins become so slim that they take away the incentive to invest in advertising to get doctors to consider prescribing it. Consequently, acarbose never sold well in the United States. However, in Europe, acarbose is a popular medication for treating diabetes.

Because acarbose has no known effects besides inactivating the enzyme that digests starch, it illustrates how effective slowing carbohydrate absorption can be for treating conditions caused by insulin resistance.

Blunting the Glucose Spike

Like acarbose, certain foods consumed with carbohydrates slow the absorption of glucose into the bloodstream. Even a small blunt of the after-meal glucose spike can have a large effect on insulin demands. Most natural carbohydrates—such as fresh fruit, vegetables, and nuts—contain plenty of natural carb blockers. Some contain physical barriers to digestion, such as the cellulose walls in fruits and vegetables. Some trigger hormones that slow stomach emptying. Others contain substances that act like acarbose, and inhibit digestive enzymes.

HOW TO SLOW CARB DIGESTION

Your digestive tract is like a conveyor belt in a factory. You put the raw material in one end and different parts of your digestive system work on it as it travels along the route. If you understand what happens at each stage of digestion, you will see several points at which you can slow this process. Let's look at the machinery that breaks down and absorbs carbohydrates as they proceed through your digestive tract and consider ways to slow the process down.

The Grinder

The first step of digestion is mastication, the process of chewing. The smaller food particles are, the faster you'll digest them and the more they will raise your blood sugar. If you prepare food al dente or slightly undercooked, so it's more chunky when you swallow it, it will take longer to digest and raise your blood sugar less. Fruit and vegetables eaten whole will raise your blood glucose less than ones that are juiced or made into smoothies. Slow the process down by:

- Serving vegetables and pasta al dente—slightly undercooked so they remain crunchy.
- Eating fruit and vegetables whole rather than blended or juiced.

The Hopper

The next stop is your stomach. Food doesn't get absorbed there; rather, your stomach acts as a hopper—a place to store food between meals and a regulator of the speed with which food passes into your intestine. If you already have food in your stomach when you eat a carbohydrate, the carbohydrate will be diluted by the other foods and pass into your intestine more slowly than if you consumed it on an empty stomach. Your stomach also gets food ready to be processed by your intestines. Muscles in your stomach walls squeeze and massage its contents, mixing food with digestive juices until it turns into a thick liquid ready for passage into your intestine. Substances that resist liquefaction, such as the fiber in fruits and vegetables or the gristle in meat, slow down this process. Mushy food gets digested faster than crispy foods do. Slow down carb absorption by:

- Including foods such as meat and vegetables that resist liquefaction at meals.
- Only eating starch or sugar with other foods, never on an empty stomach.

The Control Valve

A muscular ring called the *pyloric sphincter* functions as a valve that opens and closes the outlet of your stomach. It regulates the speed with which food leaves your stomach and passes into your intestine. This is a potent tool for controlling the speed with which your digestive system processes carbohydrates.

Your pyloric sphincter is activated by a feedback system of hormones and nerve circuits that originate in your intestine. When your intestine senses that it has as much food as it can handle, it sends a message to your pyloric valve to tighten up and slow the passage of food into your intestine. It turns out that you actually have some control over how your pyloric valve works. This provides a way for you to not only slow the absorption of carbohydrates but also control your appetite.

The most potent stimulator of your pyloric valve is the presence of fat in your intestine. As soon as fat passes through your pyloric valve and reaches your intestine, it activates a reflex that closes the pyloric valve, which keeps food from exiting the stomach. It doesn't take much fat to do this. Scientists have found that as little as 2 teaspoons (10 g) of fat before a meal will slow stomach emptying. If you eat a fatty snack—a piece of cheese or a handful of nuts—10 or 15 minutes before a meal, it will close the pyloric valve. When you sit down to eat you will still have plenty of room in your stomach to enjoy your meal. However, because the tightened pyloric valve slows the passage of food out of your stomach, it takes less food to fill you up. You'll ultimately end up eating less.

Surgeons use this principle when they perform weight loss surgery. A common procedure is to wrap an adjustable band around the stomach. This acts like a tightened pyloric valve, slowing the passage of food into the intestine. People who have had the surgery still experience hunger and enjoy eating, but they fill up faster. This type of surgery usually produces substantial weight loss and markedly improves diabetes. Tighten the pyloric valve by:

- Eating a fatty snack 10 or 15 minutes before a meal.
- Taking fish oil supplements, if you use them, 10 or 15 minutes before a meal.
- Starting your meal with a salad with an oil-based dressing.

The Disassembler

There's one more step food has to take before it can enter your bloodstream. It has to be broken down into its basic building blocks—glucose, amino acids, and fatty acids.

Your intestinal cells can't absorb starch. It has to be broken down into individual glucose molecules, which can pass through the walls of your intestine and into your bloodstream. Your intestine relies on one enzyme to do this—amylase. It is the disassembler of starch. It unhitches glucose molecules from each other and frees them up so they can be absorbed.

Vinegar inhibits amylase and has been proven to slow the absorption of starch in humans. It has been used for centuries to treat diabetes. Studies show that 2 tablespoons (30 ml) consumed before eating starch lowers the after-meal glucose and reduces demands for insulin. Vinegar doesn't have to be consumed straight. It can be sprinkled on food as a condiment—a common practice in Mediterranean countries—or used in a salad dressing.

A lot of plants contain natural amylase inhibitors. In nature, their purpose is to protect plants from being devoured by insects. For example, white beans contain an amylase inhibitor called phaseolamin, which in the 1980s was marketed as a starch blocker. Although phaseolamin inhibits amylase in the test tube, it turned out not to work so well in humans. Scientists later found that stomach acid deactivates it. Subsequently, the U.S. Food and Drug Administration made companies stop advertising it as a starch blocker.

Acarbose is similarly a natural substance produced by soil bacteria, which slows the absorption of starch and reduces blood sugar and insulin levels. It has proven effective for treating diabetes and PCOS and reduces the risk of heart disease. It also promotes weight loss and reduces blood pressure. Inhibit amylase by:

- Starting your meal with a salad with a vinegar-based dressing.
- Sprinkling vinegar on your salad, even if the dressing isn't vinegar-based.
- Using vinegar as a condiment.
- Including a pickle with your meal.
- Considering the use of acarbose.

NATURAL SPONGES FOR DIGESTIVE JUICES

When glucose molecules are unhitched from one another, they float around in your digestive juices until they come into contact with the lining of your intestine, where tiny "transporters" latch onto them and pull them into your bloodstream. You can slow the absorption of glucose by eating foods that contain fiber—the insoluble parts of fruits and vegetables—or by taking fiber supplements such as psyllium. Like a sponge, fiber soaks up digestive juices, which prevents glucose molecules from coming into contact with your intestinal lining.

Fiber is nature's most plentiful carb blocker. It is the main reason fresh fruits and vegetables don't raise your blood glucose levels as much as starch and sugar do. All fruits and vegetables contain fiber, although most vegetables contain approximately twice as much as most fruits.

Scientists have found that 10 grams of fiber can reduce after-meal blood glucose levels by as much as 20 percent. This requires eating a couple of servings of vegetables. Remember that a small reduction in the after-meal glucose level results in a large reduction in insulin demands. The table on pages 64 to 66 lists the fiber content of various fruits, vegetables, legumes, and fiber supplements, according to the U.S. Department of Agriculture's National Nutrient Database for Standard Reference. Note: Gram amounts per serving size may vary among the charts in this book, depending on the source of the information and food preparation methods.

FIBER CONTENT OF COMMON FRUITS, VEGETABLES, LEGUMES, AND FIBER SUPPLEMENTS

Food	Serving size	Fiber (grams)
Fruit		
Raspberries	1 cup (123 g)	8.0
Blackberries	1 cup (144 g)	5.3
Strawberries, sliced	1 cup (166 g)	3.3
Avocado	½ avocado (101 g)	6.7
Papaya, pieces	1 cup (145 g)	2.5
Apricot	3 apricots	2.1
Grapefruit	½ grapefruit	1.4
Watermelon, diced	1 cup (150 g)	0.6
Vegetables		
Artichoke hearts, cooked without salt	1 cup (168 g)	9.6
Sauerkraut, canned	1 cup (142 g)	4.1
Collard greens, chopped	1 cup (36 g)	1.4
Carrot, cooked without salt, sliced	1 cup (156 g)	4.7
Turnip greens, cooked without salt	1 cup (144 g)	5.0
Broccoli, chopped	1 cup (91 g)	2.4
Spinach, cooked without salt	1 cup (180 g)	4.3
Brussels sprouts	1 cup (88 g)	3.3
Okra, cooked without salt, sliced	1 cup (160 g)	4.0
Green beans	1 cup (100 g)	2.7
Cabbage, cooked without salt	1 cup (150 g)	2.8
Mushrooms, white, cooked without salt, pieces	1 cup (156 g)	3.4
Cauliflower, chopped	1 cup (107 g)	2.1
Turnips, cubed	1 cup (130 g)	2.3
Dandelion greens, chopped	1 cup (55 g)	1.9
Peppers (red bell), chopped	1 cup (149 g)	3.1
Asparagus, cooked	½ cup (90 g)	1.8

(continued)

Food	Serving size	Fiber (grams)
Onions, cooked without salt	½ cup (105 g)	1.5
Mustard greens, cooked without salt, chopped	1 cup (140 g)	2.8
Peppers (green bell), chopped	1 cup (149 g)	2.5
Scallions, chopped	½ cup (50 g)	1.3
Eggplant, cubed	1 cup (82 g)	2.5
Carrot	7.25 inch (19 cm)	2.0
Lettuce, loose leaf, shredded	2 cups (72 g)	0.9
Celery, chopped	½ cup (51 g)	0.8
Lettuce, romaine, shredded	2 cups (94 g)	2.0
Tomatoes, chopped	1 cup (180 g)	2.2
Bean sprouts (mung)	1 cup (104 g)	1.9
Water chestnuts, sliced*	1 cup (70 g)	4.0
Cucumber pickle (dill)	1 large (135 g)	1.4
Lettuce, iceberg, shredded	2 cups (144 g)	1.7
Spinach	2 cups (60 g)	1.3
Onions	¼ cup (40 g)	0.7
Lettuce, butterhead, shredded	2 cups (110 g)	1.2
Alfalfa sprouts	1 cup (33 g)	0.6
Cucumber, peeled, sliced	1 cup (119 g)	0.8
Mushrooms, sliced	1 cup (70 g)	0.7
Beans and legumes		
Lentils, cooked without salt	1 cup (198 g)	15.6
Beans, pinto, cooked without salt	1 cup (171 g)	15.4
Beans, lima, cooked without salt	1 cup (188 g)	13.2
Beans, kidney, cooked without salt	1 cup (177 g)	11.3
Chickpeas, cooked without salt	1 cup (164 g)	7.6
Beans, navy, cooked without salt	1 cup (182 g)	10.5
Peas, frozen, cooked without salt	½ cup (80 g)	3.6

(continued)

Food	Serving size	Fiber (grams)
Nuts and seeds		
Chia seeds, dried	1 oz (28.3 g)	9.8
Almonds	24 nuts (28.8 g)	3.6
Sunflower seeds, dried	¼ cup (35 g)	3.0
Hazelnuts	20 nuts (28 g)	2.7
Peanuts	1 oz (28.3 g)	2.4
Walnuts, black, dried	1 oz (28.3 g)	1.9
Cashews	1 oz (28.3 g)	0.9
Fiber supplements		
Psyllium husks*	1 tbsp (12 g)	3.0
Oat bran	¼ cup (23.5 g)	3.6
Guar gum	1 oz (28.3 g)	21.9
Metamucil*	1 tsp (5.95 g)	3.0

Source: U.S. Department of Agriculture National Nutrient Database for Standard Reference, http://ndb.nal.usda. gov/ndb/search, except those items marked by (*), which were obtained from package labels. All foods are raw unless otherwise noted. Gram amounts per serving size may vary depending on information source and food preparation methods.

Although most vegetables have low glycemic loads, beans are an exception. They're loaded with fiber, but have higher glycemic loads than other vegetables. Although they're not usually classified as refined carbohydrates like bread, potatoes, and rice are, they contain a significant amount of starch.

The high fiber content of beans slows the absorption of glucose released by other foods. However, you need to take into account the glucose released by the beans themselves. Pay attention to how they're prepared. Beans mixed in sugary sauces, such as barbecue or tomato sauce, have glycemic loads that exceed 100.

Like wheat, potatoes, and rice, beans are a cheap way to provide calories. Consequently, they are dietary staples in many parts of the world. Like other starchy staples, beans were not part of the prehistoric diet—our digestive system did not evolve to handle a lot of beans.

Chia seeds provide a pleasant way to increase the fiber content of your diet as well as improve your bowel habits. These are tasty little seeds about the size of grains of sand. Chia is frequently used in meal preparation in Latin and South America. Sprinkling a tablespoon (12 g) over a salad adds texture and can virtually double a salad's fiber content. If you have any doubts that these little seeds act like sponges, put a spoonful in the bottom of a glass and slowly add water. They swell up to about ten times their original size. Slow down the absorption by:

- Eating two servings of vegetables with any starch-containing meal—for example, a salad and a green vegetable.
- Not eating more than 1 cup (250 g) of beans at a time and no more than ½ cup (125 g) if they're served in tomato or barbecue sauce.
- Taking a fiber supplement (if you use one), such as psyllium, before the meal in your day most likely to contain starch or sugar.
- Sprinkling 1 tablespoon (12 g) of chia seeds on salads to increase their fiber content.

First Responders

Your beta cells have a special supply of insulin ready to be released at the first sign of a carb heading toward your bloodstream. This is called the first-phase insulin response. It keeps your blood glucose from rising as much as it otherwise would and reduces the total amount of insulin ultimately needed to handle a carbohydrate.

Protein, as in meat, eggs, and dairy products, enhances the first-phase insulin response. This early burst of insulin reduces the after-meal glucose spike and decreases the amount of insulin ultimately needed to handle the meal. Reduce your need for insulin by:

- Including a serving of protein with any carbohydrate-containing meal.

Escape Valve

Let's say you slipped up and had a little more starch with your meal than you should have. What to do? Get up and go for a walk. Activating your muscles opens channels in cell membranes that allow glucose to pass into your muscle cells *without the need for insulin*. This begins as soon as you start moving and stops when you stop. One way to blunt an after-meal glucose spike is to do something physical immediately following the meal. It doesn't have to be vigorous exercise; an after-meal stroll will work, or some yardwork or housework. Lower your after-meal blood glucose level by:

- Getting moving—go for a walk, clean the garage, do some housecleaning.

THE CARB-BLOCKING EFFECTS OF A CONVENTIONAL DINNER

The conventional dinner is structured as if to maximize the possibilities for carb blocking. Maybe we have a natural instinct for it.

- Sometimes we have a fatty appetizer, such as nuts, cheese, or meat, before dinner. The fat in such snacks tightens the pyloric sphincter.
- We often have a salad before dinner. The greens and vegetables contain fiber, which soaks up glucose released by starch in the intestine.
- Our salad dressings often contain vinegar, which inhibits amylase.

- The appetizer and salads are usually consumed before starch. Their presence in the stomach dilutes any starch consumed during the meal, and slows its entry into the intestine.
- We usually have a full serving of protein—meat, chicken, or fish—which enhances the first-phase insulin response.
- We save dessert for last, which ensures that all carb blockers are in place before we eat it.
- Sometimes we take a stroll after dinner, which activates insulin-independent glucose uptake.

Combining Carb Blockers

You can rev up carb blockers by combining them, which produces results that are greater than the sum of its parts. For example, the combination of fiber and vinegar is more effective than doubling either carb blocker alone. Combining several weak carb blockers can add up to a significant carb-blocking effect, which is why the glycemic load of a mixed meal is usually less than the total of the individual glycemic loads. For example, the glycemic load of a hamburger with a bun is less than that of the bun alone.

8 REMOVE BELLY FAT FIRST

If those old jeans still fit over your hips but you're having trouble buttoning them, if every pound you gain seems to go straight to the old breadbasket, you're not alone. Countless books, magazine articles, and websites proffer cures for belly fat, but the solutions they suggest are always the same—just lose weight. Obviously, if you lose enough weight you will lose fat everywhere, including your belly. But is there a way to remove fat from your abdomen first? Indeed, there is.

You can lose weight by reducing your fat intake, carbohydrate intake, or both. However, if you especially want to lose belly fat, your best bet is to cut carbohydrates. Just as excess insulin increases abdominal fat, lowering insulin levels selectively removes fat from the belly. Using body scans to measure abdominal, buttock, and thigh fat in a group of women with insulin resistance, scientists instructed one group of women to go on a low-carbohydrate diet and another group to consume the same amount of calories on a low-fat diet. The groups lost the same amount of weight, but the subjects who followed the low-carbohydrate diet lost significantly more fat in their abdomens.

BELLY-SHRINKING EFFECTS OF EXERCISE

If you're serious about shrinking your belly, don't neglect exercise. As you know, exercise reduces the amount of insulin your body produces. It will remove fat from your abdomen even if you don't lose weight. When people start exercising, they often notice a marked reduction in their waist size after losing just a few pounds (kilograms). In one study, researchers had one group of women lose weight by exercising only and another group lose the same amount of weight by dieting only. The women who lost weight by exercising lost more fat in their abdomen relative to the rest of their body than those who lost the same amount of weight by dieting alone.

As discussed in chapter 5, you don't have to sweat and strain in a gym to reduce your insulin levels; walking is enough. Researchers find that sedentary folks who start walking 45 minutes a day (about 2½ miles, or 4 km) invariably lose weight, most of it from the abdomen.

One thing you should know is that exercising your abdominal muscles won't make you lose any more fat from your belly than exercising other muscles would, just as exercising your buttock muscles won't make you lose any more weight from your buttocks than exercising other muscles would.

ESTROGEN REPLACEMENT

Research shows that the tendency for women's waists to expand when they go through menopause can be counteracted by taking estrogen replacement pills or patches. In addition to preventing the hot flashes, insomnia, and mood changes that often accompany menopause, estrogen replacement therapy helps prevent the usual increase in waist-to-hip ratio.

Estrogen has another effect on body shape. It protects against osteoporosis—a softening of the bones that occurs with aging. Osteoporosis affects women more than men, and contributes to a change in body shape that often occurs after menopause. Osteoporosis causes the lower spine to shorten, which reduces height and makes the abdomen pooch. It also causes the upper spine to bend forward, creating the so-called dowager's hump.

Estrogen replacement suffered some bad publicity when a study published in 2002 found that certain estrogen pills raised the risk of breast cancer. The increase was slight—one chance in a thousand per year—and was seen only in a group that took the hormone *progesterone* along with estrogen. (Doctors add progesterone to keep the inner lining of the uterus from building up, which increases the risk of uterine cancer.) Women who took estrogen alone actually had less breast cancer than women who took no hormones. The same study found that estrogen replacement reduced the risk of colon cancer by roughly the same amount it increased the risk of breast cancer.

Estrogen replacement also raises the risk of blood clots in the legs. The chances are approximately one in a thousand. The risk subsides after the first year of taking estrogen. This risk is nullified by regular exercise.

As much as women fear breast cancer, a bigger killer is heart disease. It is the leading cause of death of men and women and kills six times more women than breast cancer does. Before menopause, women's natural estrogen production helps protect them against heart attacks. Heart attacks are rare among nonsmoking women before menopause.

After menopause, evidence suggests that estrogen replacement may similarly protect against heart disease. It's important for women to make their decision about taking estrogen around the time of menopause and not several years later. Women who start estrogen after age sixty have an increased incidence of heart attacks in the first year of taking it. If going without estrogen for several years allows the arteries to develop atherosclerosis, estrogen replacement later may trigger a clot in a diseased artery.

Here are two situations in which estrogen replacement is especially beneficial:

- Premature menopause, such as when the ovaries stop producing estrogen or are surgically removed before the age of forty. This significantly increases the chances of heart disease and osteoporosis.
- After a hysterectomy. If the uterus has been removed, there is no need to take progesterone with estrogen to protect your uterus. Evidence suggests that taking estrogen alone actually helps protect against breast cancer as well as heart disease.

TZDS

A type of diabetes medication called thiazolidinediones (TZDs) works by moving fat out of the muscles and abdomen and back into normal fat storage areas elsewhere. Removing fat from muscles increases their responsiveness to insulin and reduces blood glucose. TZDs do not promote weight loss; in fact, they often cause a slight weight gain even as they reduce abdominal fat. The weight gain can be countered by diet and exercise as well as by taking metformin.

Although insulin-resistant individuals often have more than normal amounts of fat in their abdomens, they often have *less than normal* amounts of fat on their buttocks and thighs. TZDs help redistribute fat out of the abdomen and back to the buttocks and thighs. If you have diabetes and this kind of body fat distribution, TZDs are a logical option for controlling your blood glucose as well as shrinking your abdomen.

9 MYTH BUSTERS

The enemy of your effort to reduce your consumption of one kind of food is to waste effort trying to reduce your intake of another. At the top of the list of things that people waste effort worrying about are cholesterol and fat.

THE CHOLESTEROL MYTH

There's no doubt that high blood levels of bad cholesterol cause heart disease. If you have high blood cholesterol, you need to discuss it with your doctor. However, contrary to five decades of dietary misinformation, high blood cholesterol *does not* come from eating cholesterol-containing foods. Cholesterol is an essential component of cell membranes, hormones, and other substances essential for life. The body can't depend on dietary intake to provide cholesterol. Your liver makes most of the cholesterol in your body. If you eat less cholesterol, the liver makes more. If you eat more, it makes less. Actually, the cholesterol in food is difficult to absorb. Most of it passes through your digestive tract and out in your stool.

All animal products contain cholesterol. Most of the cholesterol in our diet comes from red meat, chicken, fish, eggs, and dairy products. Eggs contain by far the highest concentration—there's more cholesterol in an egg than in a steak. Yet the cholesterol levels of people who eat a lot of eggs are no different from those who rarely eat them. Researchers studied one man who ate between twenty-five and thirty eggs daily for years. They measured his bad cholesterol level, good cholesterol level, and cholesterol particles, among several other blood tests, and could find no ill effects. His bad cholesterol was lower than average, and his good cholesterol was higher than average. He was eighty-eight years old and had no blood vessel problems.

When researchers finally concluded that cholesterol alone in food doesn't raise blood cholesterol, they suspected it must be the combination of fat and cholesterol that causes high blood cholesterol. Most sources of cholesterol in our diet—red meat, chicken, fish, and dairy products—also contain significant amounts of fat. This was an attractive idea to those who held to the dictum that "you are what you eat." They figured you get fat from eating fat and get high cholesterol from eating cholesterol with fat. The only foods that contain both fat and cholesterol are animal products, so the idea that dietary fat and cholesterol caused these conditions suggested that two of our major health problems—obesity and heart disease—come from eating animal products. The hope was that you could lose weight and prevent heart disease by avoiding animal products; fatty vegetables, such as nuts, olives, and avocados; and vegetable oils. This notion also dovetailed with concerns about animal cruelty and preservation of the environment. However, among scientists, the notion that dietary fat and cholesterol caused heart disease was highly controversial.

Then, in the 1970s, government got involved. With no evidence that avoiding fat and cholesterol would in fact prevent heart disease or obesity, the U.S. government took it upon itself to get folks to reduce their intake of fat and cholesterol. It was the first time any government endeavored to get people to eat less of any particular food.

Well, it turns out that you really aren't what you eat. Once in your system, fat, protein, and carbohydrates are all interchangeable. Your body can change carbs to fat, fat to carbs, and protein to fat or carbs. If you eat a carbohydrate, within minutes your body will turn it into the very fat you're trying to avoid. If you try to avoid fat, you usually end up eating more refined carbohydrates and producing more insulin, which will make you fat *and* diabetic.

It takes a long time to disprove a dietary theory. Virtually all of the evidence suggesting that dietary fat and cholesterol cause heart disease came from observational studies, wherein it's impossible to separate dietary habits from other factors that influence heart attack risk. The only way to prove that changing diet in a particular way will reduce the risk of a disease is to do an interventional study: select two groups of subjects at random, get one group to make the change you want to study, and follow both groups to see whether they develop the disease in question. When it comes to studying the effects of diet on the risk of heart disease, interventional studies require a large investment of time and money, and don't always produce anticipated results.

In 2011, Walter Willett, M.D., head of the department of nutrition at the Harvard School of Public Health and a scientist who has published more scientific articles on nutrition than any other researcher in the world, addressed the annual meeting of the National Lipid Association. He said that fifteen years earlier, he would not have expected to ever say what he was about to say: that dietary fat and cholesterol are not what cause heart disease. The cover of the June 14, 2014, issue of *Time* magazine featured a picture of a slice of butter with the title, "Eat Fat" and the subtitle, "Scientists thought fat was the enemy. Why they were wrong." In March 2015, a consensus of the U.S. Food and Drug Administration's advisory committee on diet recommended lifting restrictions on dietary fat and cholesterol and focusing on reducing refined carbohydrates.

It's curious why the cholesterol myth has persisted despite so much evidence against it. A generation of Americans was raised with the belief that fat and cholesterol were bad for them. Once we become convinced that a food can make us sick, the idea of eating it evokes a gut response that's hard to counteract.

One reason the myth persisted pertains to a couple of hot-button social issues: animal cruelty and preservation of the environment. One solution would be for everyone to eat nothing but plant products. However, humans evolved to eat animal products. For millions of years, humans depended on meat as their main source of calories, protein, and other nutrients. Unlike herbivores, whose digestive systems can break down raw vegetation into fuel, humans' digestive tracts could not extract enough calories from the plant products available in prehistoric times to survive.

The dilemma of how we humans can remain healthy without being cruel to animals and despoiling the environment is yet to be solved. But the fact remains: humans evolved to eat meat. It's difficult to eliminate animal products without consuming unhealthy amounts of rapidly digestible carbohydrates and causing your body to produce excessive amounts of insulin.

What Causes High Blood Cholesterol?

In a word: genetics. The human gene pool is filled with thousands of genetic quirks that raise blood cholesterol levels—some by a little, some by a lot. Approximately 30 percent of Americans—even higher percentages in many countries—have cholesterol levels high enough to raise the risk of blood vessel blockage. Most of these defects involve the receptors in the liver that remove cholesterol from the blood.

High blood cholesterol in the absence of other risk factors, such as smoking or high blood pressure, rarely causes artery blockages before age forty. Most cave dwellers died of infections, starvation, or trauma. They lived long enough to pass their genes on but rarely long enough for cholesterol to accumulate in their arteries. As recently as a hundred years ago, the average American didn't live long enough to have to worry about heart disease. At the turn of the twentieth century, the leading causes of death were pneumonia and tuberculosis.

SALT: SHAKE OFF YOUR WORRIES

You can't live without salt. In prehistoric times, humans died for lack of it. Salt, or sodium, holds fluid in the body. Without enough salt, we lose fluid, our blood pressure falls, and our vital organs don't get enough blood. Our kidneys evolved to retrieve every last grain of salt from urine so we don't waste it. How long our ancestors could survive without food or water often depended on how well their kidneys could preserve salt.

The main concern about dietary salt is its relationship to high blood pressure. Unfortunately, as we age, our kidneys' eagerness to save us from *low* blood pressure sometimes works against us and causes *high* blood pressure. Our kidneys mistakenly sense that our blood pressure is too low and activate hormones and nerve circuits that raise it. These reflexes constrict your blood vessels, stimulate your heart, and cause your kidneys to work even harder to retrieve salt from the urine, all of which raise your blood pressure. High blood pressure can eventually damage your arteries, especially when combined with other risk factors, such as smoking, high cholesterol, diabetes, and insulin resistance.

If you have high blood pressure, you can sometimes lower it modestly by reducing your salt intake, which counteracts your kidneys' eagerness to retrieve salt from the urine. However, because other mechanisms such as heart stimulation and blood vessel constriction are in play, avoiding salt in your diet usually doesn't lower your blood pressure much. In fact, reducing salt often causes the kidneys to activate those mechanisms, which counteracts your efforts to avoid salt.

The most effective treatment for high blood pressure is diuretics, which cause the kidneys to let salt out in the urine. As more salt appears in the urine, the kidneys sense that all is well—there is no threat of low blood pressure—and stop triggering reflexes that stimulate the heart and constrict the blood vessels. Diuretics alone often lower blood pressure to normal, although additional medications are sometimes needed to relax the heart and open up the blood vessels.

Most blood pressure experts agree that if you have high blood pressure, avoiding large amounts of salt will help lower it. Although salt restriction by itself usually doesn't lower the blood pressure to normal, it sometimes reduces the amount of medication needed. However, if you are already taking a diuretic, which helps your body get rid of salt, there's little benefit from trying to avoid salt in the diet.

Will avoiding salt do you any good if you don't already have high blood pressure? There is little evidence that lowering your salt intake below average will prevent you from developing high blood pressure. In fact, some studies suggest that a lower-than-average salt intake is actually worse than an average salt intake.

Most people can eat all the salt they want, even more than average, and not develop high blood pressure. There's a saying in medicine that the dumbest kidney is smarter than the best doctor. Your kidneys can tell whether you're taking in more or less salt than you need. If you take in more, they let it out in the urine. If you reduce your salt intake, your kidneys will counteract your efforts by letting less out. The bottom line: it's debatable that avoiding salt will do you any good.

Should you try to reduce your intake anyway, just in case it might help? Reducing one's salt intake is more difficult than you might think. It's not just a matter of avoiding the saltshaker.

Table salt is a minor contributor to most people's salt intake. The main source is processed foods. In fact, the largest source of salt in the American diet is bread. To make a dent in your salt intake, you have to avoid a lot of foods. If this diverts your attention from doing what you need to do—reducing your glycemic load—then it's not worth the effort.

One thing that does help is to make sure you're getting enough of the mineral potassium, which is found in fruits and vegetables and has a slight blood-pressure–lowering effect. Fruits and vegetables are full of potassium, which may be more important in your diet than excluding sodium. The National Institutes of Health recommends eating five servings of fruits and vegetables per day.

TRANS FATS: NO WORRY FOR LOW-GLYCEMIC-LOAD EATERS

The newest dietary threat is trans fats. These are vegetable oils that have been altered by a process called partial hydrogenation to keep them from becoming rancid with storage. This extends the shelf life of packaged foods made with vegetable oil, including crackers, chips, pie crusts, and biscuits. Trans fats have a mild cholesterol-raising effect, and some researchers suspect they increase the risk of heart disease. Margarine is loaded with trans fat; real butter contains little.

The good news is, if you follow a low-glycemic-load diet, you don't have to worry about trans fats. Most of the trans fats in our diet come from margarine and partially hydrogenated oil used to make starch palatable. If you eliminate starch, you eliminate trans fat.

SILLY WASTES OF EFFORT

Just as avoiding things you think are bad for you—when they really aren't—is a waste of effort, doing things you think are good for you, but aren't, is also a waste. Here are some things we have been told will make us healthier, but really won't.

Eight Glasses of Water a Day

The fruits, vegetables, and animal products we eat contain plenty of water. You shouldn't need to force yourself to drink liquids; your natural thirst mechanisms will tell you when you need to drink. Your body has powerful mechanisms that regulate water balance. The slightest decrease in water content triggers compelling thirst and an outpouring of the hormone vasopressin, which provokes thirst and sharply reduces the amount of water that goes out in the urine.

Perhaps the notion that drinking lots of water makes you healthy comes from the belief that it washes away toxins, like pouring water over a bowl of lettuce to wash away dirt. In fact, water in excess of what you need to survive doesn't even enter your cells. You would die of water toxicity if it did. Extra water goes directly to your kidneys and out in your urine. Ironically, drinking more water than you need to maintain adequate hydration can make you prone to dehydration. Excessive water drinking reduces your kidneys' ability to retrieve water from the urine, so your body can't conserve water as well it should. Consequently, you can't go without water as long as you otherwise could.

Drinking Smoothies

The idea of concocting a mysterious brew that will unlock the key to our metabolism appeals to us. That's why scientists administer placebos to subjects when they're testing the effects of a new medication. Just doing something that gives you hope, such as taking a pill, often makes you feel better.

If drinking smoothies is the only way you're going to consume fruit and vegetables, they may do you some good. However, smoothies have higher glycemic loads than you might expect from their ingredients. There are several reasons for this. When you pulverize fruits and vegetables, you break apart cell walls and barriers, which speeds digestion. In addition, liquefied food is not as filling as solid food is, so you end up consuming more fruit and vegetables than you would if you just ate them whole. As a rule, food in liquid form causes more weight gain than food in solid form does. This is especially true of sugar-sweetened beverages, but it also pertains to fruit juices and smoothies.

Protein Bars and Shakes

These supposedly high-protein products originally marketed to bodybuilders don't have nearly as much protein as eggs, meat, or dairy products do. Knowing that muscles are mainly protein, bodybuilders figured if you ate more protein, you would build more muscle. These products weren't intended to help you lose weight. In fact, because some bodybuilders believe that loading up on carbohydrates before exercise improves performance, many of these products are high in carbohydrates. However, there is no reason to believe that they help build muscle or aid in weight loss.

10 MEDICATIONS THAT CAN HELP

Doctors use several different kinds of medications for treating insulin resistance in patients with diabetes. These can also reverse insulin resistance in folks without diabetes, but doctors rarely prescribe them for insulin resistance alone. Physicians are understandably hesitant to prescribe drugs for something that can be treated with lifestyle changes alone. Nevertheless, insulin resistance causes problems and medications that improve it can help.

In preceding chapters, I discussed natural ways you can increase the muscle's sensitivity to insulin, slow the absorption of carbohydrates, and reduce the amount of glucose in your bloodstream. The medications doctors use for treating insulin resistance work in the same way. Although none work as well as the natural approach, they can enhance it. All have been proven to be effective for treating problems caused by insulin resistance, such as obesity, type 2 diabetes, and polycystic ovary syndrome (PCOS).

METFORMIN

Although your liver is capable of manufacturing glucose, it normally doesn't produce much because you get plenty in your diet. However, if you haven't eaten for a few hours, your liver will kick into action and secrete enough glucose to keep your levels from getting too low.

When you eat carbohydrates, your liver is supposed to stop producing glucose. As soon as the glucose from the carbs you eat hits your bloodstream, your beta cells produce insulin, and one of insulin's jobs is to turn off glucose production by your liver. However, if you have insulin resistance, your liver doesn't get the message. It keeps producing glucose even though you got enough from the food you ate.

One of the most effective medications available for treating type 2 diabetes is metformin. It works by stopping the liver from overproducing glucose. You might say that it acts as an internal low-carb diet. Metformin improves virtually anything caused by insulin resistance. It is the number one medication for treating type 2 diabetes, and prevents diabetes among individuals with insulin resistance. It also restores normal menstruation and fertility in women with PCOS. Metformin promotes weight loss, reduces triglyceride levels, raises good cholesterol, and lowers blood pressure.

The proven success of metformin in treating insulin resistance is testimony to the importance of reducing the amount of glucose entering your system. You might wonder about taking metformin even though you don't have diabetes or PCOS. If you have a large belly, have a high triglyceride level, have been told you are prediabetic, or have signs of PCOS and are not making progress reversing those problems with lifestyle changes alone, in my opinion it is reasonable to take metformin.

One condition in which (in many doctors' opinions) metformin is underused is PCOS. Although PCOS is not immediately dangerous, it can have devastating effects on the lives of girls and women. Of all the problems insulin resistance causes, PCOS manifests itself the earliest in life—often in the teens or twenties. Even though metformin can be helpful in reversing this condition, it's often difficult for patients or their doctors to accept the idea of taking diabetes medication for anything other than diabetes. The hesitancy of girls and women to take metformin is such a common problem that pharmaceutical companies in Europe have started marketing candy-flavored metformin, sending a message to young folks that it isn't just for adults.

The only common side effect of metformin is diarrhea. This goes away immediately upon stopping it or reducing the dose. Metformin is eliminated by the kidneys. It doesn't harm the kidneys, but if you have weak kidneys, your body may have trouble getting rid of it. You should have a blood test to check for weak kidneys before taking it. Metformin is considered safe to use during pregnancy. In fact, there is evidence to suggest that metformin reduces the rate of miscarriages among women with PCOS.

OTHER MEDICATIONS THAT SLOW CARB ABSORPTION

Although medical science has never come up with a way to the prevent carbs from being absorbed into your bloodstream, there are medications that slow down the process. Acarbose, as discussed in "Starch-Blocking Medication" on page 60, inhibits amylase, the enzyme responsible for breaking down starch into glucose. Slowing the digestion of starch reduces the speed at which glucose enters the bloodstream. Even a modest reduction in the speed of glucose absorption significantly lowers the amount of insulin needed to metabolize it.

Acarbose has been proven effective for treating type 2 diabetes as well as preventing diabetes in people with insulin resistance. It has also been proven effective in treating PCOS. Like a low-glycemic diet, acarbose promotes weight loss, lowers triglyceride levels, raises good cholesterol, and lowers blood pressure. Several studies have found a reduced risk of heart attacks in patients randomly assigned to take acarbose.

Acarbose is safe enough that in many countries you can buy it without a prescription. It is as safe to take as any pill commonly prescribed for any condition. It doesn't even go into your bloodstream like other pills do.

By slowing the absorption of starch and making bread, potatoes, and rice behave more like fruits and vegetables, acarbose may initially cause an increase in gassiness, just as an increase in dietary fruits and vegetables would. This usually resolves in a few days.

The beauty of acarbose is that you only need to take it before eating a starch-containing meal. It's best taken immediately before starting to eat. Some of my patients keep a bottle in their kitchen and take it before eating bread, potatoes, rice, or pasta.

GLP-1 Analogues

Another medication that works by slowing carbohydrate absorption is a newer type called glucagon-like peptide-1 (GLP-1) analogues, including exenatide and liraglutide. These medications have a duel action. They slow carbohydrate absorption, like acarbose does, *and* they reduce glucose production by the liver, like metformin does.

In addition to being an effective treatment for type 2 diabetes, these drugs have a potent weight-loss-promoting effect. In 2015, the U.S. Food and Drug Administration approved liraglutide for treating obesity in people with or without diabetes.

TZDs Improve Muscle Response to Insulin

No medication can come close to exercise for increasing your muscles' responsiveness to insulin. However, thiazolidinediones (TZD), discussed in chapter 8, can help a little. As you know, when your fat cells can't hold any more fuel, they start spilling fatty acids into your bloodstream, which infiltrate your muscles, making them unresponsive to insulin. TZDs remove fat from your muscle cells, which increases their responsiveness to insulin.

TZDs are commonly used for treating diabetes. Studies show they can prevent diabetes in individuals with insulin resistance. TZDs have also been proven effective for treating PCOS, although they haven't been proven safe for women planning to become pregnant.

Unlike other drugs used to treat insulin resistance, which promote weight loss, TZDs promote modest weight gain—an average of approximately 8 pounds (3.6 kg). The weight gain can be counteracted by diet and exercise and by taking metformin, which neutralizes this effect. The increase in fat that TZDs cause is usually in areas other than the abdomen. They actually reduce abdominal fat by redistributing it to other parts of the body.

SGLT2 Inhibitors Let Glucose Leave in Urine

If your blood glucose level rises too high, glucose will spill out in your urine, which is actually a good way to get rid of excess glucose. However, your kidneys don't see it that way. They consider it wasteful. They try to retrieve all the glucose they can from the urine and put it back into your bloodstream. A protein in your kidney called sodium-glucose co-transporter-2 (SGLT2) does the work.

Doctors now have medications that inhibit SGLT2, allowing more glucose to escape in the urine. These pills help normalize blood glucose levels in patients with diabetes. By reducing the amount of glucose in the system, SGLT2 inhibitors reduce the body's demands for insulin. Like other medications that reduce insulin levels, SGLT2 inhibitors promote weight loss, an effect enhanced by loss of calories through the urine.

SGLT2 inhibitors also allow salt to escape through the urine, which has a blood-pressure-lowering effect. Sometimes patients with high blood pressure can reduce the doses of their medication. However, if the blood pressure gets too low, it can cause dizziness. Among women, glucose in the urine can sometimes trigger vaginal yeast infections.

Unlike other approaches discussed in this book for lowering insulin levels, there is no natural way to get your kidneys to let glucose out in your urine.

SHOULD YOU RESORT TO MEDICATIONS?

We all like the idea of curing health problems naturally, without the use of medications. Plus, it's hard to consider something a disease when it affects a third of the population. The signs and symptoms of insulin resistance can creep up on you over the course of years. You get used to them and take them for granted.

If insulin resistance ends up causing diabetes or PCOS, you'll probably seek treatment for it and take medication if it helps. Your willingness to take medications for insulin resistance depends on the extent to which problems like abdominal obesity, high blood pressure, cholesterol imbalance, and PCOS concern you. In my opinion, while these problems are best treated by eliminating the conditions that cause them—our starchy diet and sedentary lifestyle—if you can't make progress reversing them, it's reasonable to consider medications for relieving insulin resistance.

PART III

RECIPES AND MEAL PLANS FOR REDUCING INSULIN RESISTANCE

BY DANA CARPENDER

LOW-CARB COOKING

We hope you are convinced of the value of a low-starch, low-sugar diet for controlling and reversing insulin resistance and the disastrous results to which it leads. Carbohydrate restriction is also a great way to eat simply for abundant good health and energy. There is nothing like stable blood sugar and a functioning, fat-burning metabolism to do away with the pernicious fatigue that has become the most common health complaint. Once your body has adapted to the carbohydrate restriction, which rarely takes more than a couple of weeks, you'll have the kind of energy you haven't had since high school.

Forget all those low-fat, low-calorie diets you have suffered through. You are not going to be hungry. Just as important, you're not going to be living on dry, flavorless food. You'll be amazed at just how luxurious this way of eating is, though it can take a little adjustment. You may not be familiar with some of the ingredients. Let's start by taking a look at the replacements for sugar and flour, as well as thickeners and flavorings.

Erythritol

Of the sugar alcohols (a.k.a. polyols) that add sweetness to low-carb recipes, erythritol has the least impact on blood sugar. It is neither digested nor absorbed, but simply passes through the digestive tract. By contrast, your body absorbs roughly half of maltitol, the sugar alcohol most frequently used in commercial sugar-free sweets. And erythritol, unlike maltitol, causes virtually no gut upset. These two qualities have made it one of the sweeteners I reach for most often.

However, erythritol is harder to work with. Maltitol behaves like sugar in cooking, producing gooey caramels, silky sauces, and crunchy brittles. Erythritol melts in warm mixtures, but has a tendency to recrystallize as it cools, making the final results grainy. It also has the peculiar property of being endothermic, meaning that when it hits the moisture in your mouth, it literally absorbs energy and creates a cooling sensation. This works well in ice cream, but can be disconcerting in a cookie. Erythritol is only about 70 percent as sweet as sugar, so I usually combine it with liquid stevia, the next ingredient on our list. The food industry does, too: Truvia is a combination of erythritol and stevia.

My favorite erythritol product is Swerve, which includes oligosaccharides, a sweet-tasting fiber. Swerve measures like sugar, and because of the oligosaccharides, browns nicely. It comes in both a granular version and a powdered confectioners' style. I generally prefer the powdered because of the potential for graininess with erythritol, though I keep both versions on hand. The main drawback of Swerve is its price. Plain erythritol, though not cheap, costs around $7 per pound (455 g). I pay about $12 per pound (455 g) for Swerve.

If you cannot find erythritol locally, you can order it—along with many of the ingredients on this list—either through a health food store or online at Amazon.com and Netrition.com.

Liquid Stevia

Liquid stevia extracts in dropper bottles are far easier to use than the old-school, highly concentrated, powdered stevia, and taste much better in a variety of flavors. The ones I keep on hand and have used in this book are:

- Plain: Great for a touch of sweetness in a recipe, without other flavor overtones. I've been using NuNaturals plain liquid stevia.
- English toffee: I use this constantly. The flavor bears a similarity to brown sugar.
- Vanilla: I often add vanilla extract, as well, and combine vanilla stevia with English toffee or with other flavors.
- Chocolate: The uses are numerous, from hot cocoa to cookies.
- Lemon drop: This is good not only in lemon-flavored recipes but also in recipes with a fruit flavor.

I can buy all of these flavors and more at my local health/international/gourmet grocery. Consider NOW and SweetLeaf brands. If you're not blessed with a great local health food store, you can order these items from Amazon.com, like everything else on the planet. I checked Netrition.com and found only the plain stevia extracts, but that may change. It's worth looking again.

The recipes in this book **assume liquid stevia to be of a sweetness so that 6 drops equals 1 teaspoon (4 g) of sugar**. I start with ¼ teaspoon of stevia to replace ¼ cup (50 g) sugar, and ½ teaspoon stevia to replace ½ cup (100 g). If your liquid stevia is considerably more or less sweet than this, you will need to adjust quantities. Look at the manufacturer's website for equivalents.

Almond Meal

Almonds ground to a fine meal are sometimes labeled almond flour. Bob's Red Mill makes a good one that is widely distributed.

Flaxseed Meal

This is flaxseed ground to a fine meal. Bob's Red Mill puts out a couple of different versions; I like the Golden Flaxseed Meal.

Coconut Flour

Ground from the "meat" after the oil is pressed out, coconut flour is low in starch and very high in fiber. It also has a fairly steep learning curve, but I've included it in a recipe or two.

Vanilla Whey Protein

A few recipes call for vanilla whey protein powder. I've used several brands, and never had one not work. Designer Whey Protein is perhaps most widely available; GNC stores carry it. Recently I've been using Vitacost.com's house brand, because the price is right and it works.

Guar or Xanthan

Believe it or not, you've been eating guar and xanthan all along. They're finely milled soluble fibers that are widely used as thickeners by the food-processing industry. That's how we'll be using them, too. Instead of starchy thickeners such as flour, cornstarch, or arrowroot, we use these flavorless fibers to thicken gravies, soups, sauces, and even smoothies. They also help lend structure to baked goods that are made with nut meal instead of with wheat flour. These thickeners are far more powerful than starches. If you try to do a one-for-one substitution, the results will be suitable for surfacing roads. Trust the voice of experience.

The easiest way to use guar or xanthan (they're interchangeable) is to put it in an old salt or spice shaker, and keep it by the stove. When you have a sauce or soup that needs thickening, start whisking it *first,* then keep whisking while you sprinkle the powder lightly over the surface. Stop when your dish is slightly less thick than you want it; it will continue to thicken on standing.

Hot Sauce

I am a die-hard chili-head. A few varieties made their way into this book:
- Original Tabasco/Frank's/Louisiana brand. These are pretty much interchangeable.
- Chipotle hot sauce. Chipotle Tabasco is great, as is Melinda's Chipotle Hot Sauce. Chipotle's distinctive smoky flavor has no substitute.
- Sriracha. This red jalapeño sauce from Southeast Asia has taken the world by storm. Huy Fong, the most popular brand, is known as "rooster sauce" because of the rooster on the label.

Bouillon Concentrate

Several recipes call for bouillon concentrate. I use Better Than Bouillon, which comes in paste form in jars. Unlike many brands of granules, cubes, or liquids, it contains some beef or chicken. If you prefer, you can reduce homemade beef or chicken stock until it's syrupy, store it in the freezer, and use in place of commercial bouillon concentrate.

Spike Vege-Sal

This is a subtle, seasoned salt with powdered dried vegetables mixed in. It enhances all kinds of things, and is especially good on steak. Vege-Sal is an old-time health food brand. Modern

Products recently added the name "Spike," also the name of their flagship product, to Vege-Sal. They're not the same; the original Spike has a considerably more assertive flavor.

Tofu Shirataki

Shirataki are a traditional Japanese noodle made of fiber from a root called konjac or *konnyaku*. This is sometimes mistranslated as "yam." Because they're pretty much water and fiber, shirataki are very low in calories and carbohydrates, and completely devoid of starch.

Shirataki come in two main kinds, traditional and tofu. The traditional shirataki, made only from the konjac fiber, are translucent and kind of gelatinous, quite different from the noodles we're used to. I like them in Asian dishes, but find them odd in Western-style dishes. Tofu shirataki are made from the konjac fiber with a little tofu added. This makes them white and gives them a more tender consistency than the traditional shirataki. They're not exactly like the pasta we grew up with, but I enjoy them in many ways, from chicken noodle soup to tuna casserole to fettuccini Alfredo. They've become a staple for me.

Shirataki come already hydrated in a pouch of liquid. Here's how I prep them: Put a strainer in the sink, and dump in the noodles. You will notice that the liquid smells fishy. Do not panic. Rinse the noodles well. I also snip across mine a few times with my kitchen shears, because they're really long. Dump your drained noodles into a microwavable bowl, and microwave them on high for 2 minutes. Drain them again. Put them back in the bowl and microwave for another 2 minutes, and then drain them *again*. This gets out the excess liquid, eliminating the fishiness and preventing them from diluting your sauce. Your noodles are now ready for use.

I like House Foods brand, which I can get at my local health food co-op, but if your health food store can't get them from you, you can order them online. They'll keep for a good six months in the refrigerator, so feel free to stock up. However, freezing will make them disintegrate. Not only can you not freeze them or dishes made with them, but also you'll want to order them during the warmer months, to avoid freezing during shipping.

SNACKS AND FINGER FOODS

If I had a dime for every time I've been asked, "What can I eat for snacks?" I could afford to eat out every night. The simple answer to this question is a smaller portion of anything you'd eat for a meal: a couple of chicken wings, a hard-boiled egg, a cup of soup, that sort of thing. But that's not what people mean. They're asking, "Is there something salty and crunchy that comes in a cellophane bag that I can eat without thinking about it?"

If you've got a salty-crunchy jones, you can eat pork rinds, sunflower seeds, pumpkin seeds, and nuts of all varieties. Choose ones with no sugar added and watch out for adjectives like "honey roasted." But there is a big difference between these foods and the chips you're used to: they're filling. They're high in protein, fat, and, in the case of nuts and seeds, fiber. It's good to note that these foods are available at mini-marts and truck stops. You should have no problem finding snacks while on the road; you just have to commit to choosing them. The best place to save money on nuts and seeds, however, is at a health food store, in bulk. Sometimes finger food is called for—at parties, family game night, and celebrations. Having nutritious finger food on hand is a great help in resisting the lure of junk food. Here you will find a varied selection of pick-up nibbles great for company and you!

Snack Crack

½ cup (112 g) butter
(1 stick)

¼ cup (60 ml)
Worcestershire sauce

2½ cups (363 g) raw,
shelled sunflower seeds

2½ cups (363 g) raw, shelled
pumpkin seeds (a.k.a. pepitas)

1 cup (145 g) almonds

1 cup (120 g) walnuts

1 cup (110 g) pecans

1 cup (120 g) raw
cashew pieces

2 ounces (56 g) pork rinds,
broken up into almond-size
pieces (about 2 cups)

1 tablespoon (18 g)
seasoned salt

1½ teaspoons (3 g)
garlic powder

1 teaspoon onion powder

You want crunchy, salty, and flavorful? You got it. This amazing recipe makes a lot.

Preheat the oven to 250°F (120°C, or gas mark ½). While it's heating, put the butter in a huge roasting pan, and slide it in the oven to melt.

Remove from the oven and stir the Worcestershire into it. Now add all the seeds and nuts, and the pork rinds. Stir until everything is evenly coated with the butter mixture.

In a small dish, stir together the seasoned salt, garlic powder, and onion powder. Now sprinkle this mixture evenly over the nut and seed mixture, a teaspoon at a time, stirring each addition in before adding more. Spread everything evenly in the pan. Toast the mixture in the oven for 2 hours, stirring every 30 minutes or so.

Store in a snap-top container. If you're not having a party, you might want to divide this into a few smaller containers and freeze the extra, so it doesn't go bad on you. That would be a darned shame.

Yield: 12 cups (1200 g), or 48 servings, each with 178 Calories; 16 g Fat; 8 g Protein; 5 g Carbohydrate; 2 g Dietary Fiber; 3 g Net Carbs.

Smoky Peanuts

3 tablespoons (42 g) coconut oil

2 teaspoons salt

1 teaspoon hot smoked paprika

1 teaspoon sweet smoked paprika

1 teaspoon chili powder

½ teaspoon onion powder

½ teaspoon garlic powder

6 cups (870 g) raw, shelled peanuts

In 300 Low-Carb Slow Cooker Recipes, *I included a recipe for Smokin' Chili Peanuts. This is similar but, because it doesn't use liquid smoke, it's done faster. It's a great choice for parties.*

Preheat the oven to 350°F (180°C, or gas mark 4). Put the coconut oil in a big roasting pan, and slide it into the oven to melt.

While the oil is melting, stir together all of the spices in a bowl.

When the coconut oil has melted, remove the pan from the oven, add the peanuts, and stir until they're all evenly coated. Spread them out evenly in the pan, return to the oven, and roast for 7 minutes. Pull them out, stir, turning everything over well, smooth them back into an even layer, and give them another 7 minutes in the oven.

Keep doing this until your peanuts are lightly touched with gold. It'll probably take another 7-minute stint. Pull the pan out of the oven, sprinkle about one-third of the spice mixture over the peanuts, and stir it in. Repeat with another third of the spice mixture, and then the final third.

Put the pan back in the oven, and give the peanuts about another 7 minutes. You want them nice and golden under the spices. You can serve these warm—they're awfully good that way—or you can let them cool and store them in a snap-top container.

Yield: 6 cups (870 g), or 24 servings, each with 222 Calories; 20 g Fat; 9 g Protein; 6 g Carbohydrate; 3 g Dietary Fiber; 3 g Net Carbs.

Deviled Eggs

6 hard-boiled eggs

¼ cup (60 g) mayonnaise

2 teaspoons brown mustard or horseradish mustard

Salt, to taste

Paprika, for garnish

Everybody loves deviled eggs! I make them every time I have a party, and they never fail to vanish. These are simple and classic, but feel free to play around with them.

This is so simple! Peel your eggs (boil less-than-fresh eggs—10 days old or so—for easier peeling), and slice in half. Turn the yolks out into a mixing bowl.

Add the mayonnaise and mustard, and mash it all up with a fork. If you're like me, you'll still have some hunks of yolk. Grab a big spoon, and smash them against the side of the bowl, until your yolk mixture is smooth. Now taste it. Add a little salt if you think it needs it, and another teaspoon of mustard if you like them zingy. Spoon the yolks back into the whites.

Sprinkle them with a little paprika—hot or sweet, as you prefer—and serve them to much rejoicing. Or stash them in your fridge for your next munchy attack.

Yield: 12 servings, each with 72 Calories; 7 g Fat; 3 g Protein; trace Carbohydrate; trace Dietary Fiber; 0 g Net Carbs.

Buffalo Wings

4 pounds (1.8 kg) chicken wings, cut up (sometimes labeled "party wings")

½ cup (112 g) butter (1 stick)

½ cup (120 ml) hot sauce, such as Frank's, Louisiana, or Tabasco

Restaurant buffalo wings are commonly floured, or even breaded, before being fried in dubious oil. So unnecessary! Once you realize how easy these are, you'll make them all the time. You can doctor this up if you want—add a little cayenne if you like breathing fire, or a crushed clove of garlic if you're crazy about it. But the original hot-sauce-and-butter combo is deservedly adored. Don't forget the blue cheese dressing and celery.

Depending on the season, you can grill the wings or roast them at 375°F (190°C, or gas mark 5) for about 45 minutes. Either way, get them good and crisp.

Meanwhile, melt the butter over low heat in a pan on the stovetop and stir in the hot sauce.

When the wings are crisp and done, put them in a big mixing bowl. Pour on the sauce, and use tongs to toss until they're all coated. That's it. Set them out with a stack of napkins—or better yet, a roll of paper towels—and plates for the bones.

Yield: 28 servings, each with 107 Calories; 9 g Fat; 6 g Protein; trace Carbohydrate; trace Dietary Fiber; 0 g Net Carbs.

Bacon Cheese Crackers

12 ounces (340 g) bacon

7 ounces (196 g) fontina cheese, shredded

1½ cups (235 g) raw, shelled sunflower seeds

¼ teaspoon baking powder

½ teaspoon xanthan

½ teaspoon pepper

1 egg white

Salt, for sprinkling

Yes, Bacon Cheese Crackers. You're welcome.

Preheat the oven to 350°F (180°C, or gas mark 4).

Start cooking the bacon by your preferred method until it's crisp.

Run the fontina through the shredding disk of a food processor. Transfer to a bowl and swap out the disk for the S-blade.

Put the sunflower seeds, baking powder, xanthan, and pepper in the food processor, and process until you have a fine meal.

Break the bacon into 3- to 4-inch (7.5 to 10 cm) lengths, and feed them into the processor while it's running.

When the bacon is worked in, add the cheese, one-third at a time. When the cheese is worked in, add the egg white. Process until you have a clump of dough.

Line a cookie sheet with baking parchment. Shape one-third of the dough into a ball, and put it in the middle of the parchment. Cover with a second sheet of parchment. Now roll the dough out into as thin and even a sheet as you can. (Silicone rolling pin rings found at housewares stores or online make this much easier. Use the thinnest rings.) Peel off the top layer of parchment.

Using a thin, straight-bladed knife, score the dough into squares, triangles, or diamonds. You'll find it easier to place the whole blade edge along the line you want to cut and press down rather than to draw the blade along in a slicing motion. Sprinkle lightly with salt.

Bake for 17 to 18 minutes, or until browned. These are better a little overdone, so err on the side of another minute.

Repeat with each of the remaining two-thirds of the dough. Store in a snap-top container for 36 hours to crisp up.

Yield: 86 servings, each with 46 Calories; 4 g Fat; 2 g Protein; 1 g Carbohydrate; trace Dietary Fiber; 1 g Net Carbs.

Walnut Bread

1½ cups (180 g) walnuts, divided

3 cups (255 g) shredded coconut meat

2 teaspoons erythritol

1½ teaspoons baking soda

1 teaspoon guar or xanthan

¾ teaspoon salt

½ cup (56 g) flaxseed meal

6 drops of English toffee liquid stevia

4 eggs

½ cup (120 ml) water

1 tablespoon (15 ml) apple cider vinegar

This bread is dense and flavorful, and wonderful toasted and slathered with butter or cream cheese or both. For something elegant, toast, spread with chèvre (goat cheese), and then run it under the broiler until it melts.

Preheat the oven to 350°F (180°C, or gas mark 4). Line a loaf pan with nonstick foil.

Spread the walnuts on a shallow baking tin, put them in the oven, and set the timer for 6 minutes.

Meanwhile, put the coconut, erythritol, baking soda, guar, and salt in a food processor, and start it. Scrape down the sides every few minutes.

When the timer beeps, pull the walnuts out of the oven and add 1 cup (120 g) of them to the mixture in the food processor, then run it again. Process until the mixture has the texture of a nut butter.

Add the flax meal and run the processor, scraping down the sides once or twice, until well blended.

Add the liquid stevia and then the eggs, one by one, blending each in thoroughly before adding another.

In a glass measuring cup, combine the water and the vinegar. With the food processor running, pour this through the feed tube in 3 additions, letting each get worked in before adding more. Scrape down the sides if needed.

Once the vinegar-water is in, you need to work quickly. Add the remaining ½ cup (60 g) walnuts, and pulse a few times to chop them in; you want chunks of walnut in your finished bread.

Scrape the dough into the prepared loaf pan, distributing it evenly, and smooth the top.

Bake for 75 minutes, until it pulls away from the sides of the pan, and then turn out onto a rack to cool.

Yield: 20 servings, each with 140 Calories; 12 g Fat; 5 g Protein; 5 g Carbohydrate; 3 g Dietary Fiber; 2 g Net Carbs.

Pizza Crust

3½ ounces (98 g) pork rinds

2 cups (240 g) shredded
mozzarella cheese

¼ cup (25 g) shredded
Parmesan cheese

1 clove of garlic, crushed

½ teaspoon salt

½ teaspoon baking powder

8 ounces (227 g) cream
cheese, softened

4 eggs

RECIPE NOTE

Read the labels to find
pizza sauce with no
added sugar or corn
syrup. I like Pastorelli
brand, but Ragú
makes one (read the
labels, they make two
pizza sauces, one with
sugar, one without) as
does Muir Glen brand.

You can have pizza! Just top this with pizza sauce, cheese, and your favorite toppings and bake until golden and bubbly. You can use the crust right away, but chilling it makes it easier to handle and improves the texture a little.

If you're going to use the pizza crust dough right away, preheat the oven to 425°F (220°C, or gas mark 7) and line 2 cookie sheets with baking parchment.

Put the pork rinds in a food processor and grind them into fine crumbs. Transfer to a bowl and reserve.

Now put the mozzarella and Parmesan in a food processor, along with the garlic, salt, and baking powder, and run it until the cheese is finely ground.

Add the cream cheese, and run for 20 seconds or so. Now add the eggs, one at a time, working each one in well before adding the next.

At this point, you will have a soft and sticky mass of dough. To use it right away, divide the ball in two. Place one on a parchment-lined cookie sheet. Coat your clean hands with nonstick spray or oil, and pat/press the dough out quite thin, until you have a circle between 10 and 12 inches (25 and 30 cm) in diameter. Repeat with the second ball of dough.

If you make the dough in advance, put it in a snap-top container or plastic bag, and refrigerate for several hours. I leave mine in the fridge for 48 hours. The refrigerated dough will be stiffer and less sticky than it was straight out of the food processor.

If using right away, bake the crusts for 20 minutes, until golden. At this point, top and bake them just as you would any prepared pizza crust.

Yield: 2 thin crusts, or 16 servings, exclusive of toppings, each with 151 Calories; 12 g Fat; 10 g Protein; 1 g Carbohydrate; trace Dietary Fiber; 1 g Net Carbs.

BEVERAGES

Few lifestyle changes will benefit your health more than quitting liquid candy—and yes, that includes honey, agave nectar, organic cane sugar, and the natural sugar found in juices. Adding vitamins changes neither its essential sugariness nor its effect on your insulin levels. Fructose and agave nectar are often billed, accurately, as low-glycemic sweeteners. According to the Nutrition and Metabolism Society, they can still induce insulin resistance. Don't be fooled.

So what can you drink? Water, obviously, and there's nothing wrong with that. But I am unconvinced that water is vastly more healthful than all other drinks. Tea and coffee are both loaded with antioxidants, as are many herbal teas. I drink tea by the gallon, both hot and iced.

If you like your tea or coffee sweetened, choose stevia-based sweeteners—Truvia brand is widely distributed. Liquid stevia extract comes in small dropper bottles that fit easily in a pocket or purse. The added advantage is that you can add a flavor if you like—lemon drop–flavored liquid stevia is a natural with iced tea, while English toffee, vanilla, chocolate, and hazelnut stevia are great choices for coffee. If you're a devotee of fancy coffee drinks, scout out shops that have sugar-free coffee flavoring syrups—Starbucks generally does. If you like to make these drinks at home, DaVinci, Torani, and Monin all carry a range of sugar-free syrup flavors.

Diet soda is controversial. But if you are insulin resistant, there is little question that diet soda is a better choice than the sugary stuff. If having a diet soda or two a day lets you transition to a new, healthier way of eating, I say it's worthwhile. If you're worried about artificial sweeteners, there are now all-natural sugar-free sodas sweetened with erythritol and stevia. Zevia brand has a wide range of flavors, and is always popular when I serve it at get-togethers. Blue Sky, a health food store soda brand, also makes a natural sugar-free soda under the name Blue Sky Free.

Sparkling water is growing in popularity and is a great choice. La Croix is widely available and comes in several flavors. I get mixed-flavor flats of Ice Mountain sparkling water at my Costco. And Kroger, the biggest grocery chain in the United States, now has a house brand of sparkling water (labeled "seltzer") in several flavors. Be careful to distinguish sparkling water—which generally has a bit of flavor, but no sweetener at all—from clear sodas. Read the labels.

If you choose to drink alcohol, be wary. Unless labeled otherwise, anything that tastes sweet must be assumed to contain sugar. Even some things you don't think of as sugary, are. Tonic water, for instance, contains 20 grams of sugar per cup (235 ml)! Look for the diet stuff. You can, of course, mix alcohol with diet soda for, say, a rum and Coke. Crystal Lite and similar beverages can replace fruit juices.

Hibiscus Tea

1½ cups (90 g)
dried hibiscus flowers

6 cups (1410 ml)
boiling water

1 cup (235 ml) cold water

½ teaspoon plain or lemon
drop liquid stevia, or to taste

Fans of fruit punch will love this brilliant red drink.

This is super-simple: Put the hibiscus flowers in a heat-proof pitcher, and pour in the boiling water. Let it sit until cool.

Strain the tea, pressing all the liquid out of the flowers so as not to lose any. Pour the cold water through them to get out all the goodness and press again. Pour into a half-gallon (2 L) pitcher, add water to fill, and stir in the stevia. Chill well before serving.

Yield: 6 servings, each with 6 Calories; trace Fat; trace Protein; 2 g Carbohydrate; trace Dietary Fiber; 2 g Net Carbs.

Margarita-ita

1 shot tequila

1 tablespoon (15 ml)
lime juice

8 drops lemon drop
liquid stevia

Ice

8 ounces (235 ml)
orange sparkling water

Ita *is a Spanish suffix similar to "y" in English, indicating something small, young, or light. This is my go-to substitute for sugary margaritas.*

Put a shot of tequila in a tall glass. Add the lime juice and stevia and stir. Fill with ice and then pour in the orange sparkling water.

Yield: 1 serving, with 68 Calories; trace Fat; trace Protein; 1 g Carbohydrate; trace Dietary Fiber; 1 g Net Carbs.

Hot and Black

8 ounces (235 ml) hot brewed coffee

6 drops chocolate liquid stevia

6 drops hazelnut liquid stevia

⅛ teaspoon rum extract

Who needs sugary, overpriced coffee drinks? This has a ton of flavor. This is for you, black coffee fans, but if you want to add milk or cream, who am I to say nay?

Just mix it all up in a mug.

Yield: 1 serving, with 5 Calories; 0 g Fat; trace Protein; 1 g Carbohydrate; 0 g Dietary Fiber; 1 g Net Carbs.

....

Iced Caramel Coffee

1 quart (946 ml) good and strong brewed coffee, cooled

1 cup (235 ml) half-and-half

½ cup (120 ml) heavy cream

¼ teaspoon English toffee liquid stevia

¼ teaspoon vanilla liquid stevia

⅛ teaspoon vanilla extract

3 cups (450 g) crushed ice

⅛ teaspoon guar or xanthan (optional)

Do you know how much sugar store-bought iced coffees contain? Yikes! This will satisfy the yen without spiking your blood sugar. Top with whipped cream, if you like. Our tester, who goes by Silvernotes, says, "Very easy, nice, smooth, and creamy. I don't miss my candy coffee from that famous little coffee shop!"

Put everything in your blender and run until the ice quits rattling. That's it!

Yield: 6 servings, each with 124 Calories; 12 g Fat; 2 g Protein; 3 g Carbohydrate; 0 g Dietary Fiber; 3 g Net Carbs.

EGGS AND OTHER BREAKFAST FOODS

Fried, scrambled, boiled, microwaved, in omelets—eggs are a go-to choice for fast, easy, and filling food. What about yolks? Remember, sugar and starch are your worry, not fat and cholesterol. Virtually all the vitamins and antioxidants in an egg are in the yolk, so don't you dare throw them away. Anyway, they're the yummiest part. Keeping hard-boiled eggs in the refrigerator is a great habit. Few snacks are so satisfying; they'll keep you full for a long time. They also can turn bagged salad into a meal. As for fried eggs, I'll eat them with bacon or sausage and use them to dress up leftovers of every kind. Meatloaf, skillet supper, Cauli-rice, just about anything—I'll warm it up and top it with fried eggs.

Dana's Easy Omelet Method

If I had to choose just one skill to teach people trying to improve their diet, it would be how to make an omelet. First, have your filling ready. If you're using vegetables, you'll want to sauté them first. If you're making an omelet to use up leftovers—a great idea, by the way—warm them in the microwave and have them standing by.

The pan matters. For omelets, I recommend an 8- to 9-inch (20 to 23 cm) nonstick skillet with sloping sides. If you've been nervous about Teflon or Silverstone, take a look at the new ceramic nonstick pans. They're wonderful. Put your skillet over medium-high heat. While the skillet's heating, grab your eggs—two is the perfect number for this size pan, but one or three will work—crack them into a bowl, and beat them with a fork.

The pan is hot enough when a drop of water thrown in sizzles right away. Add a little fat and slosh it around to cover the bottom. Now pour in the eggs, all at once. They should sizzle and immediately start to set. When the bottom layer of egg is set around the edges—this should happen quite quickly—lift the edge using a spatula or fork and tip the pan to let the raw egg flow underneath. Do this all around the edges, until there's not enough raw egg to run.

Now, turn the burner to the lowest heat if you have a gas stove. If you have an electric stove, you'll need to have a "warm" burner standing by because electric elements don't cool off fast enough for this job. Put your filling on one half of the omelet, cover it, and let it sit over very low heat for a minute or two, no more. Peek and see if the raw, shiny egg is gone from the top surface. (Although you can serve it that way if you like; that's how the French prefer their omelets.)

When the omelet is done, slip a spatula under the half without the filling, and fold it over, then lift the whole thing onto a plate. This makes a single-serving omelet. I think it's a lot easier to make several individual omelets than to make one big one, and omelets are so quick to make that it's not that big a deal. That way you can customize your omelets to each individual's taste. If you're making more than two or three omelets, just keep them warm in the oven, set to its lowest heat.

Instant Eggs

2 eggs

Salt and pepper, to taste

RECIPE NOTE

To vary this, spend 15 minutes over the weekend making baggies of ham cubes, chopped scallions or chives, crumbled bacon, shredded cheese, or whatever you like.

These cook in a minute, right in their bowl.

Coat a microwavable bowl with nonstick cooking spray. Break the eggs into it and scramble them with a fork, giving them 30 strokes or so.

Microwave on high for 60 to 90 seconds, depending on the strength of your microwave and how well done you want your eggs. They'll puff up nicely!

Season with salt and pepper and eat right out of the bowl.

Yield: 1 serving, with 131 Calories; 9 g Fat; 11 g Protein; 1 g Carbohydrate; 0 g Dietary Fiber; 1 g Net Carbs.

Guac and Cheese Omelet

2 eggs

2 teaspoons (10 ml) bacon grease

1½ ounces (42 g) Monterey Jack, Cheddar, or Queso Quesadilla cheese

2 ounces (56 g) guacamole

Have you seen Wholly Guacamole in the little 2-ounce (56 g) packages with the peel-off lid? Fabulous! They make a guac-and-cheese omelet an option even when you're short on time or energy. I like chipotle hot sauce on this.

This is super easy. Just make your omelet according to Dana's Easy Omelet Method on the opposite page, layering in the cheese first, and then spreading the guacamole over that.

Yield: 1 serving, with 457 Calories; 39 g Fat; 22 g Protein; 6 g Carbohydrate; 1 g Dietary Fiber; 5 g Net Carbs.

Country Club Omelet

2 eggs

2 teaspoons bacon grease or other fat

2 ounces (56 g) turkey breast slices

4 slices of cooked bacon

½ of a medium tomato, sliced

1 small scallion, thinly sliced

1 tablespoon (14 g) mayonnaise

This is an omelet based on the ever-popular club sandwich.

Make your omelet according to Dana's Easy Omelet Method (page 100), using the bacon grease.

Layer in the turkey, bacon (whole or crumbled, up to you), tomato, and scallion. Fold and plate the omelet and top with a dollop of mayo.

Yield: 1 serving, with 535 Calories; 43 g Fat; 32 g Protein; 5 g Carbohydrate; 1 g Dietary Fiber; 4 g Net Carbs.

RECIPE NOTE

You can add a slice of Muenster, Swiss, or provolone to this, if you like.

Pepperoni Eggs

8 pepperoni slices

½ tablespoon (6 g) butter

⅛ of a medium onion, thinly sliced

3 eggs

1 teaspoon brown mustard

2 tablespoons (8 g) minced parsley

This is a good, simple way to vary scrambled eggs. You could use salami in place of the pepperoni.

Slice the pepperoni into thin slivers. Put a medium-size heavy skillet over medium-low heat, melt the butter, and throw in the pepperoni slivers. Fry them crisp, then remove to a plate.

Throw the onion in the skillet and sauté until it's soft and starting to brown, about 4 minutes.

While the onion is cooking, in a bowl, scramble the eggs with the mustard.

When the onions start to caramelize, throw in the parsley, and sauté for another minute or two. Then pour in the eggs and scramble. When they're mostly set, add the pepperoni and mix it in. Continue cooking until the eggs are set and then serve.

Yield: 1 serving, with 479 Calories; 39 g Fat; 26 g Protein; 5 g Carbohydrate; 1 g Dietary Fiber; 4 g Net Carbs.

Alpine Spring Frittata

1 pound (454 g) boneless, skinless chicken breast

2 tablespoons (28 g) butter, divided

Salt and pepper, to taste

¾ teaspoon paprika

½ cup (55 g) chopped, (60 g) slivered, or (56g) sliced almonds

1 pound (454 g) asparagus, skinny stalks, if available, ends snapped off

1 bunch of scallions, sliced

2 cups (240 g) shredded Swiss cheese, divided

6 eggs, lightly beaten

I made this with raw milk and grass-fed Swiss cheese, and it was terrific. Consider splurging for Gruyère for this dish.

Dice the chicken into ½-inch (1.3 cm) cubes.

Coat a big, heavy skillet with nonstick cooking spray and put it over medium-high heat. Melt 1 tablespoon (14 g) of the butter and sauté the chicken, stirring frequently. Season with salt, pepper, and paprika as it cooks.

Put a smaller skillet over medium-low heat, and melt the remaining 1 tablespoon (14 g) of butter. Add the almonds and sauté until golden.

Meanwhile, cut the asparagus into 1-inch (2.5 cm) lengths. Stir your chicken and almonds!

When the chicken is no longer pink, add the asparagus and scallions to the skillet and stir them in. Cook for a few minutes, just until the asparagus turns brilliant green.

Stir all but 2 tablespoons (14 g) of the almonds into the chicken mixture. Stir 1 cup (120 g) of the Swiss cheese into the chicken mixture, distributing it evenly. Turn the heat to low. Spread everything evenly in the skillet. Add the eggs to the skillet, mixing and making sure the eggs seep down to the bottom.

Sprinkle the remaining 1 cup (120 g) of cheese over the top. Cover the skillet, and cook for 15 minutes or until mostly set. Turn on the broiler and place the rack 6 to 8 inches (15 to 20 cm) below it.

Broil for 5 minutes. Now give it a quarter turn, and broil another 3 to 5 minutes, just until the cheese is golden. Pull it out and sprinkle the reserved 2 tablespoons (14 g) of almonds over the top.

Cut into wedges and serve!

Yield: 6 servings, each with 412 Calories; 27 g Fat; 37 g Protein; 6 g Carbohydrate; 2 g Dietary Fiber; 4 g Net Carbs.

Breakfast for Supper

1 pound (454 g) bulk sausage

1 small turnip

2 tablespoons (30 ml) water, divided

1 small onion

½ of a green bell pepper

6 eggs

4 ounces (112 g) Cheddar cheese, shredded

This filling egg-and-sausage dish will please the whole family. I use hot sausage.

Put a big, heavy skillet over medium heat, and start browning and crumbling the sausage.

Meanwhile, peel and dice the turnip into ¼-inch (6 mm) pieces. Put them in a bowl, add 1 tablespoon (15 ml) of the water, cover with a saucer, and microwave on high for 5 minutes.

Dice the onion and pepper. Add them to the pan when some fat has cooked out of the sausage. When the microwave beeps, drain the turnips and add them to the pan, too. Keep sautéing until all the pink is gone from the sausage.

Spread the sausage mixture evenly in the skillet. Using the back of a big spoon, press 5 evenly spaced hollows around the edge of the mixture and 1 in the center. Break an egg into each hollow.

Add the remaining 1 tablespoon (15 ml) of water to create a little steam. Scatter the cheese evenly over the whole thing. Cover the skillet, turn the heat to low, and cook until the eggs are done to your liking—mine took about 15 minutes.

Serve by scooping up each egg with the sausage mixture beneath it.

Yield: 6 servings, each with 472 Calories; 41 g Fat; 20 g Protein; 5 g Carbohydrate; 1 g Dietary Fiber; 4 g Net Carbs.

Eggs Arrabiata

2 ounces (56 g) Italian sausage

½ cup (125 g) arrabiata pasta sauce

6 olives, chopped

2 teaspoons (6 g) capers, chopped

3 eggs

2 tablespoons (10 g) grated Parmesan cheese

I simply love eggs poached in a flavorful sauce. I found Rao's brand arrabiata sauce, a spicy tomato sauce with no added sugar, to be wonderful. This is not only a great breakfast, but a quick supper, too. Read labels; Italian sausage often has sugar added. You want to check the carb count.

In a 9-inch (23 cm) skillet, preferably nonstick, over medium heat, crumble and brown the sausage.

Now add the arrabiata sauce, olives, and capers, and stir them in. Spread this all evenly in the skillet.

Crack in the eggs, cover the skillet, and turn the burner to low. Let the eggs poach until the whites are set but the yolks are still runny—maybe 5 minutes, but check at 3 or 4.

Plate the whole thing, top with the cheese, and dig in. It's amazing!

Yield: 1 serving, with 469 Calories; 37 g Fat; 29 g Protein; 4 g Carbohydrate; 1 g Dietary Fiber; 3 g Net Carbs.

RECIPE NOTE

This recipe is for one serving because I was cooking just for me, and anyway, my favorite egg skillet is 9 inches (23 cm) across. You can easily double this—just use a bigger skillet.

Quiche Crust

1½ cups (225 g) raw, shelled sunflower seeds

¾ cup (75 g) grated Parmesan cheese (use the cheap stuff in the green shaker)

¾ teaspoon salt

½ teaspoon baking powder

1 egg white

2 tablespoons (30 ml) water

Many low-carbers make crustless quiche, but I like the texture and flavor a crust offers. This basic crust will work with any quiche filling.

Preheat the oven to 350°F (180°C, or gas mark 4). Spray a 9½-inch (24 cm) deep-dish pie plate or a 10-inch (25 cm) standard depth pie plate with nonstick spray or grease well.

Put the sunflower seeds in a food processor, with the S-blade in place, and grind to a fine meal.

Add the Parmesan, salt, and baking powder, and pulse until evenly mixed.

With the processor running, add the egg white and then the water through the feed tube. You'll wind up with a soft, sticky dough.

Turn the dough out into the prepared pie plate. Use clean hands to press it into an even layer all across the bottom and up the sides. End at the rim; don't try to make a decorative edge as is often done with standard pie crust.

Bake for 15 minutes, or until it gets a touch of gold. Remove from the oven to cool. You can use this right away or make it in advance and fill later on.

Yield: 6 servings, exclusive of filling, each with 254 Calories; 21 g Fat; 13 g Protein; 7 g Carbohydrate; 4 g Dietary Fiber; 3 g Net Carbs.

Curried Cheese Quiche

8 ounces (227 g) shredded Swiss cheese

1 recipe Quiche Crust (page 107), parbaked

8 ounces (227 g) frozen broccoli, thawed

1 cup (175 g) diced turkey

½ of a medium onion, diced

2 tablespoons (28 g) butter

1 clove of garlic, crushed

2 teaspoons curry powder

5 eggs

1 cup (235 ml) half-and-half

1 teaspoon salt

Fellow food writer Diana Rattray gave me the idea to combine Swiss cheese with curry. I put my own spin on it.

Preheat the oven to 350°F (180°C, or gas mark 4).

Spread the Swiss cheese evenly over the crust. Now layer in the broccoli, turkey, and onion.

In a small skillet over low heat, melt the butter and add the garlic and curry powder. Sauté for just a minute or two.

In a bowl, beat the eggs and half-and-half together and then add the salt and butter-garlic-curry mixture. Pour this over the quiche filling.

Bake for 45 to 50 minutes, or until puffed and golden. You can serve this warm or at room temperature.

Yield: 8 servings, exclusive of crust, each with 429 Calories; 33 g Fat; 26 g Protein; 10 g Carbohydrate; 4 g Dietary Fiber; 6 g Net Carbs.

Birthday Ricotta Pancakes

1 cup (240 g) full-fat ricotta cheese

2 tablespoons (16 g) coconut flour

1 tablespoon (14 g) flaxseed meal

1 tablespoon (15 g) erythritol

¾ teaspoon baking powder

½ teaspoon salt

5 eggs

¼ teaspoon xanthan

12 drops English toffee liquid stevia

¼ cup (56 g) coconut oil

Feel free to make these on your UnBirthday!

First, put a big skillet or griddle over medium heat; you want it ready when the batter is prepared.

Measure everything but the oil into a blender, and run until you have a smooth batter.

Drip a drop or two of water onto the skillet or griddle; when it skitters around, it's hot enough. Melt a tablespoon (14 g) or so of the coconut oil on it, sloshing it around to coat the whole thing.

Now pour the batter out of the blender, into roughly 3-inch (7.5 cm) rounds. These are tender and will be easier to turn if you don't make them too big.

Fry like any pancake. Make sure they're quite done on the bottom before turning. Look for the top surface to have little holes where bubbles have burst and not filled in. Flip and cook the other side. Repeat with the remaining batter and oil.

Butter and serve with low-sugar preserves or sugar-free pancake syrup.

Yield: 16 servings, each with 89 Calories; 7 g Fat; 4 g Protein; 2 g Carbohydrate; 1 g Dietary Fiber; 1 g Net Carbs.

Hot Cereal

½ cup (73 g) raw, shelled sunflower seeds

1 cup (85 g) shredded coconut meat

1 cup (95 g) almond meal

1 cup (112 g) golden flaxseed meal

1 cup (120 g) vanilla whey protein powder

¾ teaspoon salt

Our tester, Rebecca, called this "a nice, simple option" for those cold winter mornings. Add heavy cream or half-and-half, plus a sprinkle of the sweetener of your choice.

Preheat the oven to 325°F (170°C, or gas mark 3).

Use a food processor to chop the sunflower seeds a bit. You want them about the size of a grain of rice or a little smaller.

Spread the sunflower seeds, coconut, and almond meal on a rimmed baking sheet. Toast for 8 to 10 minutes, or until just getting golden.

Dump this mixture into a big bowl and add the flaxseed meal, vanilla whey protein, and salt. Stir everything together well, then transfer to a snap-top container and store in the fridge.

To serve, put about ⅓ cup (30 g) of the cereal in a bowl and stir in ½ cup (120 ml) of boiling water. Put a saucer on top of the bowl to hold in the heat, and let it sit for 2 to 3 minutes.

Thin with a little more water to get the texture you prefer and then eat like any hot cereal.

Yield: 4½ cups (485 g), or 12 servings, each with 270 Calories; 15 g Fat; 25 g Protein; 13 g Carbohydrate; 8 g Dietary Fiber; 5 g Net Carbs.

SALADS

I urge you to make your own salad dressing. The quality of the oil used in commercial salad dressing is universally poor, and salad dressing is a snap to make. With one or two jars of homemade dressing in the fridge, all it takes is some bagged salad or a trip to the grocery store salad bar to add something green and fresh to supper. Add chicken strips, canned tuna (pop for the stuff in olive oil), chopped hard-boiled eggs, shredded cheese, or smoked salmon, and you've got a whole meal!

Italian Vinaigrette

1 cup (235 ml) extra-virgin olive oil

½ cup (120 ml) red wine vinegar

1 large or 2 small cloves of garlic, crushed

2 teaspoons dried oregano

½ teaspoon salt

¼ teaspoon pepper

This is simple, classic, and tasty.

Put everything in a clean jar, crumbling the oregano between your fingers as you add it to release the flavor. Place the lid on the jar tightly and shake like crazy. That's it! Store the jar in the fridge. When you want to use it, take it out 15 to 30 minutes beforehand to let the olive oil liquefy. Or you can put the jar in warm water. Either way, shake it again right before using.

Yield: 1½ cups (355 ml), or 12 servings, each with 162 Calories; 18 g Fat; trace Protein; 1 g Carbohydrate; trace Dietary Fiber; 1 g Net Carbs.

All-American Vinaigrette Dressing

½ cup (120 ml)
apple cider vinegar

3 tablespoons (30 g)
minced onion

⅛ teaspoon liquid stevia
(about 36 drops)

1 clove of garlic, crushed

1 teaspoon salt or Vege-Sal

½ teaspoon dry mustard

½ teaspoon pepper

1 cup (235 ml) light olive oil

My mom always made vinaigrette with apple cider vinegar; it was the only kind she had in the house. I've used wine or balsamic for years, but thought I'd try apple cider vinegar again. This is great!

Just measure everything into a clean jar, put on the lid, and shake-shake-shake. Store in the fridge; it improves overnight!

Yield: 1½ cups (355 ml), or 12 servings, each with 162 Calories; 18 g Fat; trace Protein; 1 g Carbohydrate; trace Dietary Fiber; 1 g Net Carbs.

Ranch Dressing

½ cup (120 ml) buttermilk

½ cup (120 g) sour cream

¼ cup (60 g) mayonnaise

¼ cup (25 g) sliced scallion

1 or 2 cloves of garlic, crushed

2 teaspoons lemon juice

1½ teaspoons dried dill

½ teaspoon salt

¼ teaspoon pepper

2 dashes hot sauce,
such as Tabasco or Frank's

Ranch dressing is beloved by many, but bottled varieties often have bad oils. We won't even talk about the fat-free variety, which is pretty much spicy corn syrup. This is easy, and it will get some veggies into your kids.

Simple! Assemble everything in a blender and run until it's well blended. Chill for at least a few hours for the flavors to combine.

Yield: 1½ cups (355 ml), or 12 servings, each with 63 Calories; 6 g Fat; 1 g Protein; 1 g Carbohydrate; trace Dietary Fiber; 1 g Net Carbs.

Country UnPotato Salad

½ of a large head
of cauliflower

½ cup (120 g) mayonnaise

½ cup (120 g) sour cream

2 tablespoons (30 ml)
apple cider vinegar

18 drops plain liquid stevia

1½ teaspoons (6 g)
brown mustard

2 stalks of celery, diced,
including any fresh leaves

¼ of medium red onion,
finely diced

Salt and pepper, to taste

3 hard-boiled eggs

I have many potato salad recipes that replace the potatoes with cauliflower, and they're all great. So if you have a favorite potato salad recipe, try it. If you don't, this creamy version will take that honor.

Trim the leaves and the very bottom of the stem from the cauliflower. Now cut the rest into ½-inch (1.3 cm) chunks. You want about 4 cups (400 g) of cauliflower. Steam the cauliflower until tender, about 12 to 15 minutes on high in the microwave, though you can do it on the stove top if you prefer.

While the cauliflower is cooking, make the dressing by stirring together the mayonnaise, sour cream, cider vinegar, liquid stevia, and mustard.

When the cauliflower is tender, drain it well and put it in a big mixing bowl to cool. Stirring it now and then to let out the steam will help it cool faster.

When the cauliflower is cool enough that it won't cook the other vegetables, add them and pour on the dressing. Stir until everything is evenly coated. Season with salt and pepper.

Peel and coarsely chop the eggs. Add them to the salad last, stirring them in gently, so as to keep some hunks of yolk intact.

It's nice to chill this for a few hours to let the flavors blend, but it's not essential.

Yield: 6 servings, each with 230 Calories; 22 g Fat; 5 g Protein; 5 g Carbohydrate; 2 g Dietary Fiber; 3 g Net Carbs.

Kalamata, Fennel, and Feta Salad

8 ounces (227 g) pitted kalamata olives packed in olive oil

1 fennel bulb

1 lemon, divided

6 ounces (168 g) feta cheese, cubed

¼ cup (60 ml) extra-virgin olive oil

2 tablespoons (30 ml) ouzo (optional)

2 cloves of garlic, crushed

¼ teaspoon pepper

½ of a head of cauliflower

¼ cup (15 g) minced parsley

RECIPE NOTE

Ouzo is an anise-flavored liquor from Greece. Look for it at good liquor stores.

Our tester, Rebecca, called this "very interesting for a dish that was so simple to prepare." She served it with roast chicken, and said it made the meal.

Place the olives in a nonreactive bowl (stainless steel or glass). Trim the stalks from your fennel, reserving the leaves for garnish. Halve the bulb, cut out the core, and then slice it paper-thin lengthwise. Cut across the slices a couple of times to get strips about 1½ inches (3.8 cm) long. Add them to the olives.

Scrub the lemon well, then halve it. Put one half aside, and with a very sharp, thin-bladed knife, cut the rest into teeny-weeny little dice, skin included. Pick out any seeds as you go. Add the lemon dice to the olive-fennel mixture. Add the feta to the mixture.

In a small jar, squeeze all the juice from the other lemon half. Pick out the seeds. Now add the olive oil, ouzo, garlic, and pepper. Place the lid on the jar and shake like mad. Pour this over the whole shebang, and stir gently. Refrigerate and marinate for at least 4 or 5 hours.

Trim the leaves and bottom of the stem from the cauliflower and run the rest through the shredding blade of a food processor. Steam the resulting cauli-rice until just barely tender—I give mine about 7 minutes on high in my microwave steamer. Drain it well, and let it cool.

When mealtime rolls around, stir the olive-fennel mixture into the cauli-rice, scraping every bit of marinade into the bowl. Stir in the parsley, check to see if it needs salt, and you're done.

Yield: 6 servings, each with 183 Calories; 15 g Fat; 6 g Protein; 8 g Carbohydrate; 3 g Dietary Fiber; 5 g Net Carbs.

Not Quite Tabbouleh

½ of a large head of cauliflower

1 bunch of scallions

1 small red onion

1 medium cucumber

1 bunch of parsley

1 bunch of mint

2 medium tomatoes

½ cup (120 ml) extra-virgin olive oil

¼ cup (60 ml) red wine vinegar

¼ cup (60 ml) lemon juice

Pinch of cayenne

Salt and pepper, to taste

Here's another demonstration of the versatility of cauli-rice. It stands in beautifully for cracked wheat in this recipe—a great choice for a potluck picnic.

Trim the very bottom of the stem off the cauliflower and cut off the leaves. Whack the rest into chunks, and run it through the shredding blade of a food processor. Put the resulting cauli-rice in a microwavable casserole with a lid, or better, a microwave steamer. Add a few tablespoons of water, cover, and microwave on high for 6 to 8 minutes. Don't overcook!

When the microwave beeps, uncover the cauliflower immediately! If you leave it covered, it will continue cooking. Dump the cauliflower into a big mixing bowl or salad bowl. Let it cool to the point where it won't cook the other veggies. Stirring now and then will help it cool more rapidly.

Meanwhile, slice the scallions, including the crisp part of the green shoot. Dice the red onion. Split the cuke lengthwise, scoop out the seeds, and then dice with the skin on. Mince the parsley and mint leaves. Dice up the tomatoes, too.

When the cauliflower is no more than warm, add all the other vegetables.

Now mix together the olive oil, red wine vinegar, lemon juice, and cayenne. Pour over the tabbouleh and toss the whole thing vigorously, until it's evenly mixed. Season with salt and pepper.

Refrigerate for a few hours to let the flavors blend. Toss again, to redistribute the dressing, before serving.

Yield: 8 servings, each with 153 Calories; 14 g Fat; 2 g Protein; 8 g Carbohydrate; 2 g Dietary Fiber; 6 g Net Carbs.

Green Salad with Arugula, Fennel, and Salami

3 cups (120 g)
romaine lettuce

3 cups (120 g) arugula

1 fennel bulb

1 medium tomato

¼ cup (15 g) minced parsley

2 ounces (56 g) salami, sliced
and cut into bite-size wedges

½ cup (120 ml) Italian
Vinaigrette (page 111)

*I used imported small-batch, fancy salami for this, and I think it
made a difference. Go with the best you can get.*

Tear or cut up the lettuce, and throw it in a big salad bowl with
the arugula.

Whack the stems off of the fennel. You can save some of those
pretty feathery leaves for garnish, if you like. Cut the bulb in half
lengthwise, and remove the core. Now slice it paper-thin lengthwise, and add it to the greens.

Dice the tomato, and throw it in, too, along with the parsley.

My salami was the diameter that most pepperoni is, so I sliced
it thin, then quartered those slices. That should give you an idea of
the size pieces you want. Add them, too.

Pour on the dressing, toss madly, and then serve immediately!
If you need to make this ahead of time, don't add the dressing until
the very last moment.

Yield: 6 servings, each with 141 Calories; 13 g Fat; 3 g Protein;
6 g Carbohydrate; 2 g Dietary Fiber; 4 g Net Carbs.

Simple Cucumber Salad

3 medium cucumbers

Salt, to taste

¼ of a large red onion

½ cup (120 ml) extra-virgin olive oil

⅓ cup (80 ml) white balsamic vinegar

This is super-easy if you have a food processor and not much more complicated if you don't.

Slice the cucumbers quite thin; I put mine through the thin-slicing blade of my food processor. Put these in a nonreactive bowl and sprinkle them liberally with salt—don't panic, most of it will not wind up in your salad. Toss the cukes as you salt them, so they all get salted. Let 'em sit for 15 to 20 minutes.

While the cucumbers are resting, mince the onion. Again, I did this in my food processor.

Now, using clean hands, squeeze the cucumber slices. You will discover that quite a lot of water comes out of them and the slices grow limp, yet somehow they still stay crisp. Squeeze them all quite well, then pour off the accumulated liquid.

Add the onion, olive oil, and vinegar, and stir the whole thing up. It's nice to refrigerate this for at least an hour or two before serving, but it's not essential.

Yield: 6 servings, each with 183 Calories; 18 g Fat; 1 g Protein; 6 g Carbohydrate; 1 g Dietary Fiber; 5 g Net Carbs.

RECIPE NOTE

If you'd like to drop the carb count on this a bit further, use white wine vinegar and add a few drops of plain liquid stevia.

Yankee Girl's Attempted Southern Coleslaw

½ of a head of cabbage, shredded

1 cup (120 g) very thinly sliced celery, leaves included

1 cup (240 g) mayonnaise

3 tablespoons (45 ml) apple cider vinegar

A generous ¼ teaspoon liquid stevia

½ teaspoon celery seed

I am an unregenerate Yankee with deep New Jersey roots, but I took my ideas for this from a Southern cookbook. Don't know if I got it right, but it tastes good!

Here's your basic coleslaw procedure: throw the cabbage and celery in a big mixing bowl. Mix together the mayonnaise, cider vinegar, liquid stevia (I use EZ Sweetz Stevia and Monk Fruit blend), and celery seed, pour it over the salad, and toss to coat. Let it chill for a few hours before serving.

Yield: 10 servings, each with 175 Calories; 19 g Fat; 1 g Protein; 4 g Carbohydrate; 2 g Dietary Fiber; 2 g Net Carbs.

Make-It-Yesterday Artichoke and "Rice" Salad

½ of a large head
of cauliflower

1 teaspoon chicken bouillon
concentrate

1 cup (300 g) chopped
artichoke hearts, canned
or jarred

½ of a bell pepper
(I used part green,
part orange, for color.)

3 scallions, sliced

1 stalk of celery, diced,
including any leaves

2 tablespoons (8 g) minced
parsley

⅓ cup (80 g) mayonnaise

1 tablespoon (15 ml) Italian
Vinaigrette (page 111)

¼ teaspoon curry powder

3 tablespoons (27 g)
pine nuts

Salt and pepper, to taste

This make-ahead salad will impress the family, the potluck gang, and dinner guests. Give it at least 12 hours in the refrigerator for the flavors to meld.

Trim the leaves and the very bottom of the stem from the cauliflower, cut it into chunks, and run it through the shredding blade of a food processor. Steam the cauli-rice lightly; I give it about 7 or 8 minutes on high in my microwave steamer, but you can do it on the stove if you prefer. Uncover when it's just tender, to let the steam out and avoid mushiness.

Dump the cauli-rice into a big mixing bowl. Dissolve the chicken bouillon concentrate in 1 tablespoon (15 ml) of the steaming water, and stir it into the cauli-rice. Set aside to cool.

Add the other veggies to the cooked cauli-rice mixture.

Stir together the mayonnaise, vinaigrette, and curry powder. This is, of course, your dressing. Add to the salad, and stir until everything is evenly coated.

Put a medium-size skillet over medium-low heat, add the pine nuts, and stir until they are lightly golden. Stir them into the salad. Season with salt and pepper. Chill for at least 12 hours before serving.

Yield: 6 servings, with 157 Calories; 14 g Fat; 3 g Protein; 8 g Carbohydrate; 3 g Dietary Fiber; 5 g Net Carbs.

VEGETABLE SIDES

Now that you're skipping potatoes, noodles, rice, and other starches, you may wonder what goes on the rest of the plate. Vegetables, my friend, vegetables. Don't feel you have to fancy up the vegetables if you don't care to. There's no reason not to simply steam some green beans, broccoli, asparagus, or what-have-you, and serve it with butter on top. Simple is good. They can be boiled, but the results are inferior, and nutrients are lost in the water. Different vegetables take different lengths of time to steam. Further, when I'm using frozen vegetables I generally put them in the steamer still frozen. Just read the label to make sure they don't have any starches added. I've seen vegetable blends with pasta, for example, or sugary sauces. Remember that corn is actually a grain, while peas are a legume. They're both pretty starchy. Go easy.

You can improve vast hordes of vegetables by roasting them. Asparagus, Brussels sprouts, fennel, turnips, radishes, rutabaga, cauliflower—it's hard to think of a vegetable that is *not* improved by roasting. It's simple: Preheat your oven to 450°F (230°C, or gas mark 8). Throw a few tablespoons (45 ml) of fat—olive oil, coconut oil, bacon grease, lard—in a roasting pan. (Don't use butter because it'll burn.) If you're using a solid fat, slide it into the oven for a few minutes to melt while you prep your vegetables. Toss them in the fat. Throw in a few cloves of garlic—you'll mash them after they're roasted—or some oregano, rosemary, or sage. Now roast the vegetables, stirring every 7 or 8 minutes, until they're nicely browned. Add salt and pepper, eat, and wonder why your kids are suddenly scarfing down asparagus and cauliflower and begging for more.

Fauxtatoes

½ of a large head
of cauliflower

1 ounce (28 g) cream cheese

3 tablespoons (42 g) butter

Salt and pepper, to taste

Any time you're making a main dish with a good, rich gravy, think Fauxtatoes. Do you automatically grab a sack of potatoes at the grocery store? You're going to start grabbing a head or two of cauliflower instead.

Trim the leaves and very bottom of the stem from the cauliflower and whack it into chunks. Steam until tender. I put mine in a microwave steamer and give it 12 to 14 minutes on high. If you don't have a microwave steamer, a microwavable casserole dish with a lid will work fine; just add a few tablespoons (45 ml) of water and cover. Or you can steam it on the stove. When your cauliflower is tender, drain it very well. This is essential.

Now puree the cauliflower.

Add the cream cheese and butter, and work them in. Season with salt and pepper. Serve as is, or with gravy or a little steak juice.

Yield: *3 servings, each with 159 Calories; 15 g Fat; 3 g Protein; 5 g Carbohydrate; 2 g Dietary Fiber; 3 g Net Carbs.*

RECIPE NOTE

To vary Fauxtatoes, add anything you might add to mashed potatoes.

- Sour cream and chives or scallions
- Boursin herb cheese (in place of cream cheese)
- Shredded Cheddar cheese
- Smoked Gouda or provolone
- Minced canned chipotle pepper in adobo sauce, plus a little of the sauce
- Roasted garlic, mashed
- Crisp, crumbled bacon
- Sautéed mushrooms and shredded Swiss cheese
- Pesto and chopped sun-dried tomatoes
- Horseradish

Another nice variation is to cook an equal quantity of cauliflower and celery root, also called celeriac. Just peel it, cube, and steam it until soft, and then mash it along with the cauliflower. This brings the texture closer to mashed potatoes.

Cauli-Rice

½ of a large head
of cauliflower

Here's another reason to buy cauliflower every time you're at the grocery store. Cookbook author, Fran McCullough, came up with the original idea, and I have used it a hundred ways since.

Trim the leaves and very bottom of the stem from the cauliflower, and cut it into pieces that will fit in the food processor's feed tube. Run it through the shredding blade. It should take about 5 minutes.

Steam the resulting shreds lightly. I cook mine for about 7 or 8 minutes on high in the microwave. Uncover immediately to avoid mushiness and drain well.

Yield: 4 servings, each with 18 Calories; trace Fat; 1 g Protein; 4 g Carbohydrate; 2 g Dietary Fiber; 2 g Net Carbs.

RECIPE NOTE

Here are some ways to use Cauli-Rice.

- Serve it with a main dish that has a good sauce or gravy. It's particularly nice to make a bed of cauli-rice and serve the chicken or fish, plus the sauce, right on top. It works with stir-fries, too.
- Make "seasoned rice" dishes from it: Add a teaspoon or two of bouillon concentrate, some sliced scallions or diced onion, toasted nuts, and snipped herbs. My brother John dubbed this "Rice-a-Phony," and the possibilities are endless.
- Use it in place of bulgur, couscous, or rice in grain-based salads.

Beef and Mushroom Pilaf

1 smallish or ¾ of a large head of cauliflower, leaves and bottom trimmed

3 tablespoons (42 g) butter

1 medium onion, chopped

8 ounces (227 g) sliced mushrooms

2 teaspoons beef bouillon concentrate

1½ tablespoons (23 ml) Worcestershire sauce

¼ cup (30 g) chopped walnuts

¼ cup (15 g) chopped parsley

Serve this next to a steak, or dice up leftover pot roast, stir it in, and make a skillet supper.

Cut the cauliflower into pieces that will fit in a food processor's feed tube. Run the cauliflower through the shredding blade of the processor. Put the resulting cauli-rice in a microwavable casserole with a lid, add a couple of tablespoons (30 ml) of water, cover, and microwave on high for about 5 minutes. It should be tender, not mushy.

Spray a big, heavy skillet with nonstick cooking spray and put it over medium heat. Melt the butter and start sautéing the onion and mushrooms in it. I like to break up those sliced mushrooms still further with the edge of my spatula as I sauté, but leave them in slices if you like.

When the microwave beeps, uncover the cauli-rice to keep it from cooking to a mush. When the onions are translucent and the mushrooms have softened and changed color, drain the cauli-rice and add it to the skillet. Stir everything together.

Now add the beef bouillon concentrate and the Worcestershire sauce and stir until the bouillon concentrate is dissolved and everything's coated with the seasonings. Stir in the walnuts and parsley, and serve.

Yield: 5 servings, each with 130 Calories; 11 g Fat; 3 g Protein; 7 g Carbohydrate; 2 g Dietary Fiber; 5 g Net Carbs.

Zoodles

3 small zucchini

Salt, to taste

3 tablespoons (45 ml) extra-virgin olive oil

1 clove of garlic, crushed (optional)

2 teaspoons oregano (optional)

These zucchini noodles have taken the low-carb world by storm! You'll need a spiral cutter, which you can get at any housewares store or online. Choose zucchini small enough in diameter to fit in your cutter. Serve them as you would noodles; you can simply add Parmesan, top them with no-sugar-added spaghetti sauce, or use them as a bed for a main dish with a tasty gravy—use your imagination!

Simply run your "zukes" through the spiral cutter, piling the zoodles into a mixing bowl.

Salt the zoodles, tossing as you go. Let them sit for 15 to 20 minutes.

Now use clean hands to squeeze the zoodles to get out the excess liquid, and drain well. The liquid will take much of the salt with it.

Put a big, heavy skillet over medium-high heat and add the olive oil. When it's hot, add the zoodles, tossing just until they are thoroughly good and hot. Stir in the garlic and oregano and cook for just another minute. Don't let them get mushy!

Yield: 4 servings, each with 113 Calories; 10 g Fat; 2 g Protein; 5 g Carbohydrate; 2 g Dietary Fiber; 3 g Net Carbs.

Asparagus with Browned Butter and Balsamic

¼ cup (56 g) butter

1 pound (454 g) asparagus

1½ teaspoons
balsamic vinegar

This dish is simple, yet devastatingly delicious. It's an easy recipe to double, should you have more diners.

Put the butter in a small saucepan (preferably with a good, heavy bottom) over low heat.

Snap the bottom ends off the asparagus where it wants to break naturally. Put it in a microwave steamer, or arrange spoke-fashion, tips toward the middle, on a Pyrex pie plate. Add a couple of tablespoons (30 ml) of water, cover, and cook for 3 to 5 minutes on high in the microwave, depending on how thick the spears are. You want them tender-crisp, not mushy.

Check to see if the butter has melted. Let it keep cooking until it's browned, with a nutty smell.

When the asparagus is done, drain and transfer to a serving plate. Stir the balsamic vinegar into the browned butter, then pour it over the asparagus. Yum!

Yield: 3 servings, each with 154 Calories; 15 g Fat; 2 g Protein; 4 g Carbohydrate; 2 g Dietary Fiber; 2 g Net Carbs.

Chipotle-Lime Pumpkin

14 ounces (392 g) canned pumpkin

½ cup (120 g) sour cream

1 tablespoon (15 g) canned chipotle chile in adobo sauce, minced, plus 1 or 2 teaspoons (5 or 10 ml) of the sauce

Salt and pepper, to taste

½ of a lime, cut into wedges

Everyone knows pumpkin is great in pies, but have you considered it as a savory side dish? This is easy and delicious.

Simply combine the pumpkin, sour cream, and minced chipotle in a saucepan, and heat through. Season with salt and pepper and serve with lime wedges.

Yield: 4 servings, each with 98 Calories; 6 g Fat; 2 g Protein; 10 g Carbohydrate; 3 g Dietary Fiber; 7 g Net Carbs.

RECIPE NOTE

Look for canned chipotles in adobo sauce in the international aisle, with the Mexican food. Freeze the remainder in a snap-top container.

Eric's Birthday "Mac" and Cheese

½ of a head of cauliflower

8 ounces (227 g) Cheddar cheese, half sharp, half extra-sharp, shredded

1 cup (235 ml) heavy cream

3 eggs

1 teaspoon dry mustard

½ teaspoon salt or Vege-Sal

¼ teaspoon pepper

This is so cheesy good, no one's going to care that it's cauliflower instead of macaroni.

Preheat the oven to 350°F (180°C, or gas mark 4). Grease a 3-quart (2.7 L) casserole.

Trim the leaves and the very bottom of the stem off your cauliflower. Now cut the rest into bits about ½ inch (1.3 cm) or so.

Mix the two kinds of shredded Cheddar together. Set aside ½ cup (60 g), and layer the rest in the casserole dish, starting with the cauliflower.

Whisk together the cream, eggs, mustard, salt, and pepper, and pour it over the cauliflower and cheese. Sprinkle the reserved ½ cup (60 g) of cheese over the top.

Bake for 45 to 50 minutes, or until the cauliflower is tender.

Yield: 6 servings, each with 323 Calories; 29 g Fat; 13 g Protein; 2 g Carbohydrate; trace Dietary Fiber; 2 g Net Carbs.

Upscale Green Beans

1 pound (454 g) green beans
(I use fresh, but frozen will
work, too.)

3 tablespoons (42 g) butter,
divided

¼ cup (30 g) slivered almonds

1 shallot, minced

1 clove of garlic, crushed

Salt and pepper, to taste

I've always loved beans almondine: green beans with butter-toasted almonds. This is a notch above those, and it's easy to double or triple.

Trim the tips and tails of your green beans, if needed. (My grocery store sells fresh beans already tipped and tailed, which is great.) Steam them until tender but not mushy—I gave mine 12 minutes on high in my microwave steamer.

Meanwhile, put a big, heavy skillet over medium-low heat. Add 1½ tablespoons (21 g) of the butter and let it melt. Add the almonds and stir until they're golden. Remove the almonds to a plate and reserve.

Melt the remaining 1½ tablespoons (21 g) of butter and sauté the shallot and garlic gently until softened.

When the beans are tender, drain off the excess water. Add them to the skillet along with the almonds and toss everything together. Sauté for just a few more minutes to meld the flavors. Season with salt and pepper.

Yield: 4 servings, each with 163 Calories; 13 g Fat; 4 g Protein; 9 g Carbohydrate; 4 g Dietary Fiber; 5 g Net Carbs.

SEAFOOD

If you're pressed for time, fish is your best friend. It's hard to find a fish recipe that takes more than 30 minutes, and most are done far faster. However, if you're used to breading and frying your fish, or buying it that way, you'll need some new ideas. You'll find them here.

When you need to keep it simple, consider the virtues of canned tuna (pay the higher price for the good stuff, canned in olive oil); frozen, precooked, and peeled shrimp; and smoked salmon. All of these can be great friends when your schedule is packed. About those shrimp: spike no-sugar-added ketchup (Heinz makes one) with lemon juice, a little horseradish, and a shot of hot sauce, and you've got cocktail sauce for an instant supper. And any of these make a great addition to a salad, whether bagged or from the grocery store salad bar. You'll also find grilled fish fillets with a variety of seasonings in the freezer case. Just look next to the breaded fish.

One warning: skip the fake seafood. It virtually always has added sugar or starch or both. Be wary of deli "crab" salad and the like. If it's affordable, it's probably not real crab.

Orange-Pepper Salmon

24 ounces (680 g) salmon
fillet, cut into 4 pieces

Salt, to taste

½ scant teaspoon pepper,
plus more for sprinkling on
the fish

¼ cup (56 g) butter

¼ cup (60 ml) lemon juice

16 drops of orange extract

12 drops of lemon drop
liquid stevia

Lemon and lime are often used with fish, but the orange flavor goes wonderfully with the richness of salmon.

Season the salmon lightly on both sides with salt and pepper.

Put a skillet, preferably nonstick, over medium-high heat and melt the butter. Throw in the salmon, skin-side down. Give it about 4 minutes, flip it, and give it another 4 minutes or so. How long will depend on the thickness of your fillets. While the fish is cooking, stir together the lemon juice, orange extract, stevia, and pepper.

When the salmon is done to your liking, transfer it to a serving plate. Now pour the lemon juice mixture into the hot skillet and stir it around, scraping up all the nice brown stuff. Let this simmer for a minute or two, then pour over the fish and serve immediately.

Yield: 4 servings, each with 304 Calories; 17 g Fat; 34 g Protein; 1 g Carbohydrate; trace Dietary Fiber; 1 g Net Carbs.

Cod with Tomatoes, Olives, Capers, and Feta

24 ounces (680 g) cod fillet, cut into 4 fillets

2 tablespoons (30 ml) extra-virgin olive oil

Salt and pepper, to taste

2 small tomatoes, diced

4 tablespoons (30 g) chopped olives

4 tablespoons (40 g) diced red onion

8 teaspoons (24 g) chopped capers

4 tablespoons (38 g) crumbled feta cheese

8 teaspoons (5 g) minced parsley

Add a big tossed salad and a bottle of wine, and you've got a great quick supper.

Preheat the oven to 350°F (180°C, or gas mark 4). Grease 4 gratin dishes, if you have them, or a Pyrex baking dish if you don't.

Brush each fillet with the olive oil, and season with salt and pepper on both sides. Lay them in the prepared dishes or baking dish.

Now layer the rest of the ingredients on top of the fish in the order given.

Bake for 10 to 15 minutes, or until flaky all the way through. If you've used gratin dishes, just serve them as is. If you used a Pyrex baking dish, you'll want to put the fish on serving plates, scooping out any stray bits of yumminess that have escaped and dividing them among the servings.

Yield: 4 servings, each with 254 Calories; 11 g Fat; 32 g Protein; 5 g Carbohydrate; 1 g Dietary Fiber; 4 g Net Carbs.

RECIPE NOTE

Gratin dishes are quite useful and great for baking individual servings of fish, eggs, or baked fruit. They're worth having on hand.

Sweet and Smoky Salmon

1 teaspoon hot
smoked paprika

½ teaspoon cumin

½ teaspoon salt

24 ounces (680 g) salmon
fillet, cut into 4 pieces

2 tablespoons (28 g) butter

12 drops of English toffee
liquid stevia

These are quick, easy, and beguilingly different.

In a small dish, mix together the paprika, cumin, and salt. Sprinkle this mixture evenly over both sides of the salmon fillets.

Put a big, heavy skillet, preferably nonstick, over medium-low heat. Melt the butter and stir in the liquid stevia. Add the salmon and sauté until done, about 4 to 5 minutes per side, depending on thickness. Transfer to plates and scrape every last drop of that seasoned butter over each serving!

Yield: 4 servings, each with 251 Calories; 12 g Fat; 34 g Protein; trace Carbohydrate; trace Dietary Fiber; 0 g Net Carbs.

RECIPE NOTE

If you're fond of cilantro, I think a little minced herb over each fillet would go well here.

Tequila-Lime Shrimp

2 tablespoons (28 g) lard or coconut oil

1 pound (454 g) shrimp, peeled

1 clove of garlic, crushed

½ teaspoon cumin

1½ tablespoons (23 ml) lime juice

1 tablespoon (15 ml) tequila

2 dashes of hot sauce, or to taste

Salt and pepper, to taste

This super-quick recipe will make you feel like you're eating at a beachfront restaurant in Cozumel. Don't write me asking for a substitute for the tequila because there isn't one. If you need to omit it, just have lime shrimp.

Put your biggest skillet over medium heat and melt the lard. Add the shrimp and sauté for about 3 minutes per side, depending on how big the shrimp are, until they're pink all the way through.

Stir in the garlic, cumin, lime juice, tequila, and hot sauce. Cook for another minute or two, stirring often. Season with salt and pepper, and you're done!

Yield: 3 servings, each with 253 Calories; 11 g Fat; 31 g Protein; 2 g Carbohydrate; trace Dietary Fiber; 2 g Net Carbs.

RECIPE NOTE

If you want to take an extra 15 to 20 minutes, you can brine the shrimp: Dissolve a couple of tablespoons (36 g) of sea salt in a quart (940 ml) of water, and soak the shrimp in it. The salt water is drawn into the cells, plumping the shrimp and seasoning them internally. This is a nice way to thaw frozen shrimp. Drain and pat them dry with paper towels before sautéing, or you'll have a major splatter disaster on your hands!

Cross-Cultural Shrimp

1 tablespoon (28 g) coconut oil

1 pound (454 g) shrimp, peeled

¼ cup (40 g) diced red onion

¼ cup (40 g) oil-packed sun-dried tomatoes, chopped

2 teaspoons hot sauce or sriracha

½ teaspoon dark sesame oil

½ teaspoon pesto sauce

With notes of both Europe and Southeast Asia, these shrimp have a mixed pedigree. Like most seafood, they're quick to cook. Serve them as is or over a bed of Cauli-Rice (page 122) or tofu shirataki angel hair (page 87).

Put a big, heavy skillet over medium-high. Melt the coconut oil, slosh it around, and throw in the shrimp and onion. Sauté, stirring and turning everything over frequently, until the shrimp are pink through, and then add everything else. Stir it up, let it cook for another minute or two, and serve.

Yield: *3 servings, each with 235 Calories; 10 g Fat; 31 g Protein; 5 g Carbohydrate; 1 g Dietary Fiber; 4 g Net Carbs.*

Easy Herbed Scallops

1 pound (454 g) scallops

1 teaspoon seasoned salt
(I use Real Salt brand)

½ teaspoon dried oregano

½ teaspoon dried thyme

½ scant teaspoon lemon
pepper

1½ tablespoons (21 g) butter

1½ tablespoons (23 ml)
olive oil

2 tablespoons (30 ml)
dry white wine

2 tablespoons (30 ml)
lemon juice

2 tablespoons (8 g)
minced parsley

I did this with big, impressive (and expensive) sea scallops, but you can also use bay scallops.

Drain any liquid off the scallops, and pat them thoroughly dry with paper towels. They won't sear otherwise, so get them good and dry.

Mix together the seasoned salt, oregano, thyme, and lemon pepper. Sprinkle the scallops lightly on both sides with this mixture.

Put a big, nonstick skillet over medium-high heat and add the butter and olive oil, swirling them together as the butter melts. Let this get hot before you add the scallops. Allow the scallops to brown a bit on both sides, until done—mine took about 3 minutes per side, but some were done before others.

When they're nicely golden, add the wine and lemon juice to the skillet. Swirl them about a bit with the scallops, and let the mixture cook down about halfway, until starting to get a little syrupy. Transfer the scallops to serving plates and scrape all the pan juices over them. Sprinkle a little parsley over the top of each serving, and you're done.

Yield: 2 servings, each with 386 Calories; 20 g Fat; 38 g Protein; 8 g Carbohydrate; 1 g Dietary Fiber; 7 g Net Carbs.

POULTRY

Whole chickens are often inexpensive. They take an hour or so to roast, with very little effort. And they please both light and dark meat fans. If you've got an hour to get supper on the table, you could do far worse. Vary them with sprinkle-on seasonings—Creole seasoning one day, barbecue rub another, or jerk seasoning next week. Marinate a whole chicken in olive oil and lemon juice, with garlic and oregano, before roasting, and you've got Greek chicken. I do mine in a large zip-top bag if the chicken's not too big. Otherwise, I do it in a nonreactive bowl or pan—glass, enamel, or stainless steel. Rub the marinade all over it, and turn it over every hour or two. (With a bag, you don't have to be quite so assiduous.) There's a good chance you'll have leftovers to transform into chicken salad.

Chicken Fajitas

1 pound (454 g) boneless, skinless chicken breast

1 green bell pepper

1 small onion

1 small tomato

1 tablespoon (14 g) lard

2 teaspoons lime juice

1 teaspoon chili powder

½ teaspoon cumin

½ teaspoon salt

¼ teaspoon pepper

1 clove of garlic, crushed

This dish is so good and versatile! Make a fajita salad, fill an omelet, or just dump them in a bowl and scarf them down. I add guacamole and sour cream!

Cut the chicken into ¼-inch (6 mm) strips—this is easier if it's half-frozen. Whack the pepper in half and then in half the other way. Remove the core and seeds and then cut into ¼-inch (6 mm) strips. Halve the onion end to end, and slice that way again, ¼-inch (6 mm) thick. The tomato gets the same treatment: Cut it into wedges about ¼-inch (6 mm) thick.

Put a big, heavy skillet over high heat. When it's hot, melt the lard and throw in the chicken. Sauté, stirring often. While it's cooking, stir in all the seasonings.

When all the pink is gone from the chicken, use a spatula to remove it to a plate, leaving as much of the accumulated liquid in the skillet as possible. Put the pan back over the heat and add the bell pepper and onion. Sauté until they're just starting to soften. Add the tomato and sauté until the onion is translucent.

Stir the chicken back in and use a rubber scraper to rescue all the juices from the plate. Voilà! You have achieved chicken fajitas.

Yield: *3* servings, each with 257 Calories; 9 g Fat; 35 g Protein; 9 g Carbohydrate; 2 g Dietary Fiber; 7 g Net Carbs.

RECIPE NOTE

The serving count assumes that you're serving this in bowls or on a salad. In omelets, it'll fill 4 or 5.

Cola Chicken

5 pounds (2270 g) chicken pieces, bone in, skin on

12 ounces (355 ml) diet cola, sweetened with erythritol and stevia

¼ cup (60 g) no-sugar-added ketchup (Heinz makes this.)

1 clove of garlic, crushed

1 tablespoon (15 ml) hot sauce or sriracha

3 tablespoons (45 ml) soy sauce

This super-simple slow cooker recipe depends on using diet soda sweetened with erythritol and stevia, not aspartame or sucralose. I use Zevia. Blue Sky Free is another such brand.

Plunk the chicken in the slow cooker. Mix together everything else, and pour it over the chicken. Cover the slow cooker, set it to low, and let it go for 6 hours.

When it's done, pull the chicken out and arrange it on a broiler rack. Arrange the oven rack on the second level down from the broiler, turn it on, and slide the chicken under it.

While the chicken is browning just a bit, ladle the sauce into a nonreactive pan and put it over medium-high heat. Let it reduce until it gets syrupy. During this time, you'll want to turn the broiler pan so the chicken browns evenly.

Obviously, you'll serve the chicken with the sauce! Don't forget plenty of napkins.

Yield: 8 servings, each with 424 Calories; 29 g Fat; 36 g Protein; 1 g Carbohydrate; trace Dietary Fiber; 1 g Net Carbs.

Masala Chicken

4 chicken thighs, bone in, skin on

3 tablespoons (45 ml) lemon juice

1 tablespoon (15 g) erythritol

1 clove of garlic, crushed

½ teaspoon grated ginger root

½ teaspoon red pepper flakes

3 drops English toffee liquid stevia

½ teaspoon salt

2 tablespoons (2 g) minced cilantro (optional)

This sweet-and-tangy lemon chicken has an Indian accent, and is super simple to make.

Put the chicken in an 8 × 8-inch (20 × 20 cm) Pyrex baking dish. Mix together the lemon juice, erythritol, garlic, ginger, red pepper flakes, stevia, and salt and pour it over the chicken. Turn each piece a couple of times to coat. Let this marinate for at least 45 minutes—better yet, do this first thing in the morning and let it marinate all day.

When dinnertime comes, turn on the broiler. Arrange all the thighs bone-side up. Now broil for 15 minutes. Turn the pan 90 degrees to ensure even cooking, and give it another 15 minutes.

Use tongs to turn the chicken skin-side up. This time, broil for 10 minutes before turning the pan. Baste with the pan juices and give it another 5 to 10 minutes. You don't want to scorch it. Serve with the pan juices spooned over it and the cilantro sprinkled on top.

Yield: 4 servings, each with 203 Calories; 14 g Fat; 16 g Protein; 1 g Carbohydrate; trace Dietary Fiber; 1 g Net Carbs.

Killer Chicken and "Rice"

½ of a head of cauliflower

4 chicken thighs, bone in, skin on

¼ cup (60 g) Boursin cheese

8 ounces (227 g) mushrooms, coarsely chopped

2 tablespoons (20 g) packed sun-dried tomatoes, minced

2 tablespoons (20 g) minced shallot

1 ounce (28 g) bacon, minced

Amazing! I mean, look at that ingredient list! How could it be tastier? And the cauli-rice cooks along with the chicken.

Preheat the oven to 350°F (180°C, or gas mark 4). Grease an 8 × 8-inch (20 × 20 cm) baking dish, or coat with nonstick cooking spray.

Trim the very bottom of the stem and the leaves from the cauliflower, whack it into chunks, and run it through the shredding blade of a food processor. Dump it into the prepared baking dish, and spread it into an even bed.

Use your fingers to loosen the skin on the chicken thighs. Work 1 tablespoon (15 g) of Boursin up under the skin of each thigh, and use your fingers to spread it evenly under the skin. Place the chicken on the bed of cauli-rice.

Sprinkle the mushrooms, tomatoes, shallot, and bacon evenly over both the chicken and the cauli-rice.

Bake for 50 to 60 minutes, or until the juices run clear when you pierce a thigh to the bone. The timing will depend a bit on the size of the thighs.

When done, transfer the thighs to a plate and stir the cauli-rice, blending the juices and bits of mushroom, tomato, and such into it.

Make beds of the cauli-rice on 4 plates, and nestle a thigh down into each. Done!

Yield: 4 servings, each with 342 Calories; 25 g Fat; 22 g Protein; 8 g Carbohydrate; 3 g Dietary Fiber; 5 g Net Carbs.

Kickin' Chicken Florentine

2 teaspoons hot
smoked paprika

½ teaspoon salt

¼ teaspoon pepper

4 chicken thighs,
bone in, skin on

2 tablespoons (28 g)
butter, divided

2 cloves of garlic, crushed

½ cup (120 ml) chicken broth

¼ cup (60 ml) cream

1 tablespoon (15 ml)
lemon juice

2 tablespoons (10 g)
grated Parmesan cheese,
plus more for sprinkling

½ teaspoon thyme

Guar or xanthan

10 ounces (280 g) frozen
chopped spinach, thawed,
drained, and squeezed dry

This is similar to the Chicken Florentine in my first book, but the hot smoked paprika gives it a whole new twist. Don't panic at this list of ingredients—this recipe is quite simple.

Preheat the oven to 400°F (200°C, or gas mark 6). Mix together the paprika, salt, and pepper, and sprinkle this mixture liberally on all sides of the chicken.

Put a big, heavy skillet (preferably ovenproof; cast iron is ideal) over medium heat. Melt 1 tablespoon (14 g) of the butter. When the pan is hot, add the chicken and brown it on both sides.

Transfer the chicken to a plate for a moment. Melt the remaining 1 tablespoon (14 g) of butter and sauté the garlic for a minute or so.

Now add the broth, cream, lemon juice, Parmesan, and thyme. Stir this up and let it simmer for a minute or two. Use guar or xanthan to thicken this sauce to about the texture of half-and-half.

Stir in the spinach. Get it well acquainted with the sauce. Now spread the mixture evenly in the skillet, and nestle the thighs down in it.

Transfer the skillet to the oven and bake for 40 minutes. Serve the chicken on a bed of the spinach, with a little extra Parmesan sprinkled on top.

Yield: 4 servings, each with 326 Calories; 25 g Fat; 21 g Protein; 5 g Carbohydrate; 3 g Dietary Fiber; 2 g Net Carbs.

RECIPE NOTE

If you'd like more vegetables, a bed of cauli-rice, with the spinach and then the chicken on top, would be lovely.

Turkey Skillet Supper

¼ cup (56 g) coconut oil
or lard, divided

1 pound (454 g) ground turkey

½ of a medium onion

3 cloves of garlic, crushed

12 ounces (340 g) broccoslaw

1½ teaspoons grated
ginger root

⅓ cup (80 ml) soy sauce

This is another quick and easy, one-dish meal. I used a pound (454 g) of ground turkey, but there's no reason you couldn't use diced leftover roast turkey instead. Just skip the step where you brown and crumble the turkey.

Put a big, heavy skillet over medium heat, add 1 tablespoon (14 g) of the coconut oil and start browning and crumbling the turkey. When it's about half-cooked, stir in the onion and garlic and keep cooking until all the pink is gone from the turkey.

Add the remaining 3 tablespoons (42 g) of coconut oil to the skillet and stir in the broccoslaw, ginger, and soy sauce. Stir it all up well. Now cover the skillet, turn the burner to low, and let the whole thing cook for 10 minutes. Stir, re-cover, and give it another 10 minutes. Now nibble a broccoli shred. Is it tender? If so, it's done. If not, give it another 5 minutes or so; it shouldn't take much longer than that.

Yield: 4 servings, each with 323 Calories; 23 g Fat; 23 g Protein; 7 g Carbohydrate; 2 g Dietary Fiber; 5 g Net Carbs.

RECIPE NOTE

If you're using leftover turkey, start sautéing the onion and garlic for a few minutes. Then stir in everything else, including the diced turkey, and go from there.

Turkey-Bacon-Rutabaga Hash

1½ pounds (680 g) rutabaga (about ½ of a large one)

4 ounces (112 g) bacon

½ of a medium onion

¼ cup (60 ml) bacon grease

3 cups (420 g) diced turkey (I use half dark meat, half white meat.)

Salt and pepper, to taste

Oh, yum! What a great way to use up holiday leftovers, whether with fried eggs or alone, for breakfast or supper.

Peel the rutabaga. Cut into ½-inch (1.3 cm) dice—you'll want a good, big, sharp knife for this—and put it in a microwavable casserole with a lid or a microwave steamer. Add a little water, and cook on high for 12 to 15 minutes.

In the meantime, chop the bacon, or just use your kitchen shears to snip it into a big, heavy skillet over medium-low heat. Fry the bacon bits crisp, stirring from time to time.

While the bacon's cooking, go ahead and dice the onion. When the bacon is crisp, scoop out the bits and reserve on a plate. Leave the grease in the skillet. Throw the onion into the bacon grease and start sautéing.

When the microwave beeps and the rutabaga is al dente, drain it and add it to the skillet, too. Stir it up with the onion and chop the cubes of rutabaga into smaller bits with the spatula. Keep sautéing the veggies, turning it all over every few minutes. Add more bacon grease as needed, a tablespoon (15 ml) or so at a time.

When the rutabaga starts to brown, stir in the turkey. Keep sautéing, adding more grease as needed, and turning everything over every few minutes. When it's nice and brown, with some crispy bits, season with salt and pepper. Stir in the reserved bacon bits and serve.

Yield: 4 servings, each with 513 Calories; 34 g Fat; 35 g Protein; 15 g Carbohydrate; 5 g Dietary Fiber; 10 g Net Carbs.

RECIPE NOTE

If you want to put a fried egg or two on each serving, you could get 5, maybe 6, servings out of this.

BEEF

As long as you skip the potato, bun, or other starch, dig into that red meat with gusto! Grass-fed beef is nutritionally superior to conventionally raised beef, but even the grocery store brand is highly nutritious. It's a great source of vitamin B_{12}, and a good source of B_6, zinc, iron, and, surprisingly, potassium.

The most common form of beef is the hamburger. But how to cook one perfectly? And, more perplexing, what to do with it if you're not putting it on a bun? Let me recommend the fork, a wonderful gadget that allows you to transfer food to your mouth tidily without the use of an edible napkin. Or you can do like some of the cooler burger joints and wrap your burger in several layers of iceberg lettuce. Pick up some no-sugar-added ketchup; Heinz makes a great one. (The mustard and dill pickle chips are low carb to begin with.)

Making burgers too thick forces you to overcook the outside to get the middle done. I've started making my burgers ½ inch (1.3 cm) thick, increasing the diameter rather than the thickness if I want a larger portion—or, as so many restaurants do, doubling up the patties. Cook the burger quickly—I do mine in a searing-hot iron skillet—for just 3 to 4 minutes per side. This gives you a nice, browned surface with a light pink and juicy interior. Now for some things to put on that perfect patty. If you're bored with ketchup, see the following recipes.

Bleu Burgers

Three 6-ounce (168 g each) hamburger patties

3 tablespoons (24 g) crumbled Gorgonzola cheese

1 tablespoon (10 g) finely minced red onion

Back before you could buy no-sugar-added ketchup, I hit on this and still haven't improved on it.

Cook the burgers according to the directions on page 144. During the last minute of cooking, top each with 1 tablespoon (8 g) of crumbled Gorgonzola and cover the skillet with a tilted lid.

After you transfer the burgers to plates, top each with 1 teaspoon of minced red onion.

Yield: 3 servings, each with 426 Calories; 33 g Fat; 28 g Protein; trace Carbohydrate; trace Dietary Fiber; 0 g Net Carbs.

Mushroom-and-Swiss Burgers

1½ pounds (680 g) ground chuck, made into 4 patties

2 tablespoons (28 g) butter

8 ounces (227 g) sliced mushrooms

¼ teaspoon onion powder

¼ teaspoon Worcestershire sauce

Salt and pepper, to taste

4 slices of Swiss cheese (4 ounces [112 g] total)

With all this flavor going on, who can possibly miss the bun?

Make your burgers according to the directions on page 144.

While they're cooking, put another skillet over medium heat and melt the butter in it. Sauté the mushrooms until softened and then stir in the onion powder and Worcestershire sauce. Add the salt and pepper.

When you flip the burgers, top each with a slice of Swiss cheese. For the last minute of cooking, cover the skillet with a tilted lid, leaving it open a crack.

Transfer the burgers to plates and divide the mushrooms among them.

Yield: 4 servings, each with 622 Calories; 49 g Fat; 39 g Protein; 4 g Carbohydrate; 1 g Dietary Fiber; 3 g Net Carbs.

Feta, Olive, and Tomato Burgers

1½ pounds (680 g) ground chuck, made into 4 burgers

4 tablespoons (60 g) olive tapenade

4 tablespoons (40 g) crumbled feta cheese

2 tablespoons (20 g) oil-packed sun-dried tomatoes, sliced (Buy 'em that way!)

So good! And with purchased tapenade, crumbled feta, and chopped sun-dried tomatoes, this is no more trouble than adding cheese, a pickle, lettuce, and tomato. Try this with ground lamb, too.

Make your burgers according to the directions on page 144.

After you've flipped the burgers, spread 1 tablespoon (15 g) of the tapenade on each, then add 1 tablespoon (10 g) of the crumbled feta. Cover the skillet with a tilted lid during the last minute of cooking.

Transfer your burgers to plates and top each with ½ tablespoon (5 g) of sun-dried tomatoes before serving.

Yield: 4 servings, each with 432 Calories; 34 g Fat; 28 g Protein; 1 g Carbohydrate; Trace Dietary Fiber; 1 g Net Carbs.

RECIPE NOTE

Tapenade is a highly flavorful paste of olives, capers, and seasonings. Look for it with pickles and relishes.

Hero of the Cookout Chuck Steak

⅓ cup (80 ml) lemon juice

¼ cup (60 ml) olive oil

¼ of a small onion

1 tablespoon (8 g) chili powder

1 tablespoon (15 ml) soy sauce

1 clove of garlic

1-inch (2.5 cm) piece of ginger root, a chunk about the size of a walnut, peeled

1 teaspoon meat tenderizer

3 pounds (1362 g) beef chuck roast, 1½ inches (3.8 cm) thick

RECIPE NOTE

The carb and calorie counts are high, but you won't consume all the marinade.

Chuck is inexpensive and flavorful, but tough. Marinated right, though, it's perfect for grilling. You can impress a cookout crowd without breaking the bank.

Put everything but the chuck in a food processor and process until the onion, garlic, and ginger root are pulverized.

Lay the chuck on a plate or cutting board, and stab it all over with a fork on both sides. You don't want more than ¼ inch (6 mm) between stab wounds.

Put the chuck in a gallon-size (3.7 L) resealable bag. Pour in the marinade and then seal the bag, pressing out the air. Turn the whole thing over several times, to make sure it's all coated. Toss this in the fridge for at least 8 hours; overnight is great.

When cooking time comes, drain the marinade into a bowl. Grill close to well-ashed charcoal until it's good and brown, probably 4 to 5 minutes, basting once or twice. Flip and repeat.

Now raise the grill rack or lower the firebox, whichever works for your grill, until it's as far from the fire as it can get. Close the lid and let it go another 6 minutes. Baste, flip, and give it another 6 minutes. These times are approximate, because I can't know how hot your grill is, nor how well done you like your steak. Don't baste during the last 5 minutes or so of cooking; you don't want raw meat germs on your steak.

Transfer to a platter and let it rest for 5 minutes before carving and serving.

Yield: 8 servings, each with 431 Calories; 34 g Fat; 27 g Protein; 4 g Carbohydrate; 1 g Dietary Fiber; 3 g Net Carbs.

Italian Meatballs

1½ pounds (680 g) ground beef

⅔ cup (65 g) grated Parmesan cheese

1 ounce (28 g) pork rinds, crushed into crumbs

⅓ cup (80 ml) heavy cream

⅓ cup (20 g) minced parsley

3 cloves of garlic, crushed

1 egg

½ teaspoon salt

2½ cups (625 g) no-sugar-added pasta sauce

2½ cups (590 ml) low-sodium beef broth

Serve this classic with any no-sugar-added pasta sauce. You can serve them over tofu shirataki noodles (page 87) or Zoodles (page 124), or just eat the meatballs and sauce with a sprinkle of Parmesan.

Preheat the oven to 425°F (220°C, or gas mark 7). Line a big baking pan with foil.

Now perform your basic meatball procedure: Dump the beef, cheese, pork rinds, cream, parsley, garlic, egg, and salt into a big bowl and use clean hands to squish everything together really well. Form the mixture into 15 balls, arranging them in the foil-lined pan as you go.

Bake for 15 minutes. Remove from the oven and transfer to a large, nonreactive saucepan.

Combine the pasta sauce and broth and pour over the meatballs. Bring to a simmer over medium heat. Turn the heat down to maintain a simmer, and let cook for 20 to 30 minutes, or until the sauce has reduced and thickened up again.

Yield: 5 servings, each with 646 Calories; 49 g Fat; 39 g Protein; 12 g Carbohydrate; 3 g Dietary Fiber; 9 g Net Carbs.

Salvage Stroganoff

1 pound (454 g) beef round, mechanically tenderized

¼ cup (56 g) bacon grease, divided

½ of a small onion, diced

8 ounces (227 g) mushrooms, sliced

½ cup (120 ml) beef broth

¼ cup (60 ml) dry white wine

1½ tablespoons (23 ml) Worcestershire sauce

1 tablespoon (16 g) tomato paste

1 cup (240 g) sour cream

Salt and pepper, to taste

My freezer coughed up a too-old piece of tenderized grass-fed beef round, not a cut to get excited about. This preparation turned it into a very tasty meal. It would be even better with somewhat less antiquated meat. It would also work nicely with ground chuck.

Cut the meat into strips. Put a big, heavy skillet over high heat and add 1 tablespoon (14 g) of the bacon grease. Start about one-third of the meat browning. Transfer the strips to a plate as they brown, adding more beef and more bacon grease as needed; I use 3 tablespoons (42 g) to sear all the beef strips.

When all your beef is brown and on the plate, turn the heat under the skillet to medium, melt the remaining 1 tablespoon (14 g) of bacon grease, and throw in the onion and mushrooms. Sauté together until the onion is translucent.

Add the beef back to the skillet, along with the broth, wine, Worcestershire, and tomato paste. Stir it all up. Now turn the heat to low, cover the skillet, and let it simmer for 30 minutes.

Whisk in the sour cream; after this, do not let the mixture boil, or it will crack. Season with salt and pepper to taste.

Yield: 4 servings, each with 516 Calories; 40 g Fat; 28 g Protein; 9 g Carbohydrate; 1 g Dietary Fiber; 8 g Net Carbs.

RECIPE NOTE

The classical way to serve this is over noodles—fettuccini-width tofu shirataki (page 87) would be great, here. It's also wonderful over Fauxtatoes (page 121), or just in a bowl by itself. And don't forget: leftovers are good in an omelet.

PORK AND LAMB

Owing to societal fat-phobia, some of the tastiest cuts of pork are also the cheapest. Pork shoulder, butt (really a shoulder), and picnic are consistently affordable, and ribs are often inexpensive, too. Pork is a great source of not just protein but also niacin and potassium.

Processed pork products, especially ham, call for a little caution. They virtually always have sugar added. I have seen ham with 1 gram of sugar per serving and with 5 grams of sugar per serving. That's a 500 percent difference!

I also adore lamb, but it's pricier than pork. Once or twice a year, I buy a leg when they're on sale, and have the Nice Meat Guys slice it into steaks for me, then bag 'em and stash 'em in the freezer. These are meatier than lamb chops, and far cheaper. They also come with a nice little bonus of marrow in the bone. Marrow is yummy: it's like meat butter.

Pork and Cabbage Supper

1 pound (454 g)
pork shoulder, ½ inch
(1.3 cm) thick

2 tablespoons (28 g) lard
or bacon grease

1 small onion, diced

½ of a large head of
cabbage, coarsely chopped

1 tablespoon (11 g)
brown mustard

1 tablespoon (15 ml)
apple cider vinegar

½ teaspoon celery seed

1 teaspoon caraway seed

From humble pork shoulder and cabbage comes this tasty Middle European skillet supper. Quick, easy, cheap, delicious—what more could you ask from a recipe?

Cut the pork shoulder into strips; this is easier if it's half-frozen.

Put a big, heavy skillet over medium heat, melt the lard, and add the pork. Sauté, stirring often, until the pink is gone, approximately 5 to 7 minutes.

Stir in everything else, getting it all well incorporated. Cover the skillet with a tilted lid to let the steam escape. Let it cook for 5 minutes. Stir it up again, turning everything over.

Re-cover with the tilted lid, and let it all cook for another 5 minutes. Stir it up again, give it 5 more minutes, and it's done.

Yield: 3 servings, each with 406 Calories; 30 g Fat; 23 g Protein; 13 g Carbohydrate; 5 g Dietary Fiber; 8 g Net Carbs.

Marsala Pork

3½ pounds (1590 g)
country-style pork ribs

Salt and pepper

1 tablespoon (14 g) butter

1 tablespoon (15 ml) olive oil

8 ounces (227 g) sliced white
or cremini mushrooms

6 cloves of garlic, crushed

¼ cup (60 ml) Marsala wine

¼ cup (60 ml) chicken broth

2 tablespoons (3 g) rosemary

10 juniper berries

They may be called "country-style ribs," but this recipe is down-right sophisticated. This is another case of an inexpensive cut becoming a knock-your-socks off dish.

Season the pork on both sides with salt and pepper.

Put a big, heavy skillet over high heat and melt the butter with the olive oil, swirling them together. Brown the pork on both sides. Transfer the pork to a plate.

Add the mushrooms to the skillet, turning the heat down to medium. Sauté for about 5 minutes, until they soften and change color. Scoop them onto the plate with the pork.

Drain the fat from the skillet, and put the skillet back on the heat, turning it to low.

Add the garlic, Marsala, chicken broth, rosemary, and juniper berries, and stir it all around, scraping the brown stuff up off the bottom of the pan.

Put the pork back in the skillet, and place the mushrooms around it. Cover the skillet, and let the whole thing simmer for an hour.

Yield: 6 servings, each with 497 Calories; 38 g Fat; 32 g Protein; 4 g Carbohydrate; 1 g Dietary Fiber; 3 g Net Carbs.

Simply Saucy Pulled Pork

3 pounds (1362 g) pork shoulder

2 cups (480 g) salsa

36 drops English toffee stevia

1½ tablespoons (23 g) erythritol

2 tablespoons (22 g) brown mustard

This slow cooker pork dish cooks in its own sauce.

Couldn't be easier: Plunk the pork shoulder in your slow cooker, fatty-side up.

Mix together everything else and pour evenly over the pork. Cover, set to low, and let it go for 6 to 8 hours. Use two forks to shred the pork into the sauce before serving.

Yield: 8 servings, each with 321 Calories; 23 g Fat; 23 g Protein; 4 g Carbohydrate; 1 g Dietary Fiber; 3 g Net Carbs.

Creamy, Cheesy, Ham Casserole

2 pounds (908 g) daikon (Japanese radish)

1 tablespoon (15 ml) bacon grease

½ of a medium onion, diced

½ of a medium green bell pepper, diced

3 cups (450 g) ½-inch (1.3 cm) ham cubes

3 cups (300 g) frozen green beans, cut crosswise, thawed

2 teaspoons (8 g) brown mustard

1 recipe Cheesy Chicken Soup (page 159)

1 cup (120 g) shredded Cheddar cheese

Okay, this is some work. On the other hand, it uses up leftover ham, can be assembled in advance and baked later, and is a one-dish meal the whole family will love.

Preheat the oven to 350°F (180°C, or gas mark 4). Coat a 3-quart (2.7 L) casserole with nonstick cooking spray or grease it well.

Peel the daikon, cut it into ½-inch (1.3 cm) slices, then cut the slices into cubes. Put them in a saucepan, cover with water, and bring to a boil over high heat. Cook for just 5 minutes, then drain.

Melt the bacon grease in a medium-size skillet over medium-low heat, and sauté the onion and bell pepper until they're softened and the onion is translucent, about 5 minutes.

Dump the daikon, onion, bell pepper, ham, and green beans into the prepared casserole dish. Use a spoon to stir them all up.

Whisk the mustard into the Cheesy Chicken Soup, and ladle it carefully into the casserole. Take a spoon and push things aside a bit to make sure the soup gets all the way to the bottom of the casserole dish. Scatter the cheese evenly over the top.

Bake, uncovered, for 1 hour, till golden. Let it cool for 10 minutes before serving.

Yield: 6 servings, each with 480 Calories; 36 g Fat; 27 g Protein; 14 g Carbohydrate; 5 g Dietary Fiber; 9 g Net Carbs.

RECIPE NOTE

Daikon cooks up quite mild and potato-y. If you don't have leftover ham, use deli ham. Just have the deli slice it ½ inch (1.3 cm) thick; cutting it in ½-inch (1.3 cm) cubes will be a snap. You can substitute another vegetable for the green beans; broccoli would be good, or possibly asparagus, though if you use asparagus I'd probably go with fresh, cut into 1-inch (2.5 cm) lengths.

Balti Lamb Steak

1 pound (454 g)
lamb leg steak

Salt and pepper

1 tablespoon (14 g)
coconut oil

1 clove of garlic, crushed

¼ teaspoon cumin

¼ teaspoon ground coriander

¼ teaspoon red pepper flakes

¼ teaspoon garam masala
(an Indian spice blend)

2 teaspoons (10 ml)
lemon juice

1 teaspoon tomato sauce

¼ cup (60 g) sour cream

1 tablespoon (1 g) minced
cilantro (optional)

The recipe I adapted this from was for a much more complicated tikka-style dish. It works beautifully as a simple sauce and is lick-the-plate delicious.

Put a big, heavy skillet over medium heat. While it warms, season your lamb steak on both sides with salt and pepper.

Melt the coconut oil in the skillet and throw in your lamb steak. Cook to your liking—I give my ½-inch (1.3 cm) thick lamb steaks about 6 or 7 minutes per side. Transfer the lamb to a plate and keep it warm. Turn the heat down to medium-low.

Add the garlic and let it sauté for just a minute. Now add the cumin, coriander, red pepper flakes, and garam masala. Sauté the spices, stirring constantly, for just another minute.

Add the lemon juice, tomato sauce, and sour cream and stir until you have a smooth sauce.

Divide the steak into 2 portions, top with the sauce and cilantro, and serve immediately.

Yield: 2 servings, each with 539 Calories; 43 g Fat; 33 g Protein; 3 g Carbohydrate; trace Dietary Fiber; 3 g Net Carbs.

Chili-Lemon Lamb

1 pound (454 g)
lamb leg steak

Salt and pepper

½ teaspoon
chili-lemon powder

1 tablespoon (15 ml)
olive oil

1 clove of garlic, crushed

1 tablespoon (15 ml)
dry white wine

1 tablespoon (15 ml)
lemon juice

1 teaspoon oregano

5 olives, pitted and chopped

So there I was, browsing the spice department of my beloved Sahara Mart, when "chili with lemon" jumped out at me. I grabbed it and took it home. This is the first thing I did with it. If you can't find it, just use ground red chile (not the blended chili powder used for chili con carne), and grate in some peel from your lemon.

Season both sides of the lamb steak with salt and pepper and sprinkle with the chili-lemon powder. Let that sit while you put a big, heavy skillet over medium heat.

When it's hot, pour in the olive oil and slosh it about. Throw in the lamb steak and give it 6 to 7 minutes per side, until nice and brown on both sides and still faintly pink in the middle. Transfer to a platter. Put the skillet back over the heat.

Add the garlic to the skillet and sauté for just a minute. Now add the wine, lemon juice, and oregano. Stir it all up, scraping up all the nice brown stuff from the skillet. Let this mixture cook down a little, then stir in the olives. Turn the heat to quite low.

Cut the lamb into 2 portions, divide the sauce and olives between them, and serve immediately.

Yield: 2 servings, each with 498 Calories; 39 g Fat; 32 g Protein; 3 g Carbohydrate; 1 g Dietary Fiber; 2 g Net Carbs.

RECIPE NOTE

I don't care if you use black olives, green olives, or, as I did, a combination. Just make sure they're good and strong, not the super-mild black olives that come in cans.

SOUP

Soup is soothing, warming, and homey. Sadly, it is also too often full of noodles, rice, potatoes, or other starches. I urge you to make your own broth when possible. Bone broth is among the most valuable of foods, and if you save bones you would otherwise have thrown away, it's just about free. By the way, you can save steak bones, too, and make beef broth.

Anytime you cook chicken, bring home a rotisserie chicken, or make hot wings or whatever, save the bones in a plastic bag in the freezer; I use a plastic grocery sack. Don't worry if the bones are picked clean. There is still tremendous flavor and nutrition in them, as you will see. If you have some onion trimmings, celery ends, or carrot tops, throw them in, too. (Not too many celery leaves. They get bitter.)

When you have a sack full of bones, dump them into a stockpot or a big slow cooker. Cover them with water. Add about a teaspoon (6 g) of salt and a few tablespoons (45 ml) of vinegar. Bring it to just below a simmer, and let it cook for 24 to 36 hours. (This is where a slow cooker comes in handy; you can leave it going while you're at work or asleep.) Let your broth cool, strain it into a colander, and use right away or freeze for future use.

If you'd like it to take up less space, put the strained broth back into the stockpot or slow cooker, and simmer it without a lid to reduce it by half or more. You can reduce it until it's syrupy, and use it in place of packaged bouillon concentrate. It will be very low carb and loaded with gelatin and calcium, both nutritionally valuable.

These instructions work for a turkey carcass, too, with one caveat: if your turkey is large, you will probably not be able to submerge the carcass in your stockpot or slow cooker. You'll need to simmer the bottom part of it for a while, then flip it and simmer the other end. Then you can break it up and simmer until done. I generally reduce the resulting broth by at least a third.

I do occasionally use packaged broth or stock. I generally buy Kitchen Basics, widely available in grocery stores, or Kirkland Organic, from Costco. I'm so used to homemade broth that these are a little frail-flavored for me. I generally reduce them by at least a third before using them, to improve the flavor. I just boil them hard until they cook down to my liking.

Now, a few things to do with your broth!

Cheesy Chicken Soup

3 cups (705 ml)
chicken broth

4 ounces (112 g)
cream cheese

1 teaspoon chicken bouillon
granules or paste

Guar or xanthan

4 ounces (112 g)
shredded Cheddar cheese

Salt or Vege-Sal and pepper

This started out as a sauce for a ham casserole I was making, but I quickly found that it was quite good enough to serve all on its own. A great way to get some bone broth into your diet!

In a medium-size saucepan, combine the broth and cream cheese. Put it over medium heat, and bring it to a simmer. Use a whisk to break up the cream cheese into little bits.

If you have a stick blender, switch over to it. If not, you'll just have to keep whisking. Immerse the blender and mix in the cream cheese until it's completely smooth. Blend in the bouillon concentrate.

Now use your guar or xanthan shaker to thicken the soup to the texture of heavy cream. Keep blending, and add the shredded cheese a few tablespoons at a time, making sure each addition is well blended in before adding more. Season with salt and pepper to taste, and serve.

Yield: 3 servings, each with 324 Calories; 27 g Fat; 17 g Protein; 3 g Carbohydrate; 0 g Dietary Fiber; 3 g Net Carbs.

Creamy Italian Chicken Vegetable Soup

3 quarts (2.7 L) high-quality chicken broth

1 leek

1 medium turnip

1 fennel bulb, top removed

1 bunch of kale

4 boneless, skinless chicken thighs

3 cloves of garlic, crushed

1 tablespoon (18 g) ground McCormick Mediterranean Sea Salt

¾ teaspoon red pepper flakes, or to taste

2 teaspoons Italian seasoning

1 pint (470 ml) heavy cream

RECIPE NOTE

You can prep this the night before and stash the crockery insert from the slow cooker in the refrigerator. Come morning, slip it into the base and set it for low or high, as you prefer. Note that starting with chilled soup will add a couple of hours to the cooking time.

This involves a fair amount of chopping, but it can be done well in advance. And with all those vegetables, this is a complete meal in itself.

Pour the broth into a slow cooker; I use my 5-quart (4.5 L). Turn the slow cooker to high and let the broth warm while you prepare the vegetables.

Cut the dark green leaves and the root from the leek. Slice the white part into quarters lengthwise and give it a rinse in case any dirt lurks between the layers. Now slice crosswise, about ⅛ inch (3 mm) thick. Add to the slow cooker.

Peel the turnip and cut in ½-inch (1.3 cm) dice. Into the slow cooker it goes!

Halve the fennel bulb, trim the bottom, and cut out the core. Now slice it very thinly, and cut those slices into 1-inch (2.5 cm) lengths. Add it to the rest.

Rinse the kale. Lay it on your cutting board and slice across the bunch at ½-inch (1.3 cm) intervals, then chop in the other direction, rendering your kale into little bits. Add it to the soup.

Now cut the chicken into ½-inch (1.3 cm) cubes (this is easier if it's half-frozen). You know where they go!

Add the garlic and Mediterranean seasoning to the soup along with the red pepper flakes and Italian seasoning.

Okay, give it a good stir. Now slap the lid on the pot, and decide whether you want soup within 4 hours or in 8 hours or so. This will determine whether you leave your pot on high or turn it to low.

Either way, when the veggies are tender, stir in the cream. Let the soup cook for another 10 to 15 minutes, then serve.

Yield: 6 servings, each with 428 Calories; 34 g Fat; 18 g Protein; 12 g Carbohydrate; 2 g Dietary Fiber; 10 g Net Carbs.

Cheddar-Cauliflower Soup

1 quart (940 ml) chicken broth

¼ cup (30 g) finely diced celery

2 tablespoons (20 g) minced onion

2 tablespoons (16 g) minced carrot

½ of a head of cauliflower, chopped into ¼- to ½-inch (6 mm to 1.3 cm) pieces

2 cups (470 ml) heavy cream

2 ounces (56 g) cream cheese

8 ounces (227 g) sharp Cheddar cheese, shredded

1 tablespoon (11 g) horseradish mustard

2 teaspoons seasoned salt

Guar or xanthan (optional)

How can you not like a soup that's basically cauliflower in cheese sauce?

Put the chicken broth in a nice big pan and place it over medium-low heat.

Add the celery, onion, carrot, and cauliflower. Bring to a simmer and cook until the cauliflower is tender, 20 to 30 minutes.

Stir in the cream.

Cut the cream cheese into small chunks and add them to the soup. Now whisk in the Cheddar cheese, a handful at a time, making sure each addition is melted before adding more.

Whisk in the horseradish mustard and seasoned salt. Thicken a little with your guar shaker if you like, check to see if it needs a little more seasoned salt, and you're done.

Yield: About 2½ quarts (2.3 L), 6 servings, each with 503 Calories; 46 g Fat; 16 g Protein; 7 g Carbohydrate; 2 g Dietary Fiber, 5 g Net Carbs.

Tex-Mex Turkey Pumpkin Soup

2 tablespoons (28 g) coconut oil

1 large onion, diced

4 cloves of garlic, crushed

1 cup (150 g) diced bell pepper (I used red and orange)

3 quarts (2.7 L) turkey broth (page 158)

1 can (28 ounces, or 784 g) tomatoes with green chiles, undrained

1 can (14 ounces, or 392 g) pumpkin

1½ tablespoons (12 g) chili powder

1½ tablespoons (6 g) oregano

1½ tablespoons (10 g) cumin

3 cups (525 g) diced turkey

¼ cup (15 g) minced parsley

¼ cup (4 g) minced cilantro, plus more if desired

4 avocados

8 ounces (227 g) Monterey Jack cheese, shredded

A turkey carcass yields so much good broth and meat that it's a shame to throw it away. My mom always boiled hers up with the leftover gravy and stuffing, and added some rice. Once I stopped eating bread stuffing and rice, I had to get creative. This savory one-dish meal takes advantage of the canned pumpkin that's always on sale around the holidays. For this recipe, we'll take it that you have already boiled up your carcass for soup (see the instructions for chicken bone broth on page 158), let it cool, and picked off the meat.

In a big soup kettle, over medium-low heat, melt the coconut oil and start sautéing the onion, garlic, and pepper. Let them cook, stirring often, until the onion is soft and translucent, about 5 minutes.

Add the broth, canned tomatoes, pumpkin, chili powder, oregano, and cumin. Bring to a simmer, and let it cook for 20 to 30 minutes.

Stir in the turkey, parsley, and cilantro. Bring back to a simmer, and let it go just another 5 to 10 minutes. Meanwhile, peel, pit, and dice half an avocado for each serving. If you're fond of cilantro, mince a bit more of that, too.

Ladle out the soup. Top each bowl with the shredded cheese, diced avocado, and cilantro. Serve! You don't need another single thing with this.

Yield: 8 servings, each with 431 Calories; 32 g Fat; 23 g Protein; 19 g Carbohydrate; 6 g Dietary Fiber; 13 g Net Carbs.

SAUCES

The array of jarred cooking sauces in the grocery stores has burgeoned in the past couple of decades, and with good reason. Sauces are cookery magic. They can transform leftovers, get the kids to eat vegetables, or jazz up burgers or chicken. Many of these sauces are loaded with cornstarch, flour, corn syrup, and other ingredients that are not doing your body any favors. These sauces, on the other hand, will add big flavor to your food without messing with your blood sugar. All of them can be made in advance, too, and stashed in the fridge for a few days, to make your life easier and your meals more interesting.

I'll mention here that America's favorite sauce/condiment, ketchup, is very high in sugar. A couple of teaspoons won't torpedo your plan, but you sure don't want to use ½ cup (120 g) in your meatloaf. Fortunately, Heinz, the undisputed king of the ketchup world, makes an excellent no-sugar-added ketchup. Let it be your new staple. Barbecue sauce is even more sugary than ketchup. You might as well pour pancake syrup on your ribs.

Cheese Sauce

¾ cup (180 ml) heavy cream

8 ounces (227 g) Cheddar cheese, shredded

⅓ cup (55 g) whipped cream cheese

½ teaspoon dry mustard

The trick to this sauce is to keep the heat low and add the cheese very gradually. It's great on broccoli or cauliflower, of course! Or you can add it to tofu shirataki (page 87) to make mac and cheese.

Pour the cream into a heavy-bottomed saucepan over low heat and let it slowly come to just below a simmer.

Whisk in the cheeses a bit at a time; alternate a handful of Cheddar with a tablespoon (10 g) of cream cheese, whisking until the cheese is completely melted in before adding more.

Whisk in the mustard, and you're done.

Yield: 6 servings, each with 286 Calories; 27 g Fat; 10 g Protein; 2 g Carbohydrate; trace Dietary Fiber; 2 g Net Carbs.

Kansas City-Style Barbecue Sauce

¼ cup (56 g) butter

½ cup (80 g) chopped onion

2 cloves of garlic, crushed

2 cups (480 g) no-sugar-added ketchup

⅓ cup (80 g) erythritol

¼ cup (60 ml) Worcestershire sauce

2 tablespoons (30 ml) lemon juice

2 tablespoons (40 g) blackstrap molasses

2 tablespoons (16 g) chili powder

2 tablespoons (30 ml) white vinegar

2 teaspoons black pepper

½ teaspoon salt

¼ teaspoon English toffee liquid stevia

This makes plenty, keeps well in the fridge, and—this is important—has that great Kansas City barbecue flavor. And it has less than half the sugar of standard barbecue sauce; your body, as well as your palate, will thank you.

Melt the butter in a nonreactive saucepan over low heat. Add the onion and garlic and sauté gently, not letting them brown, until the onion is soft, about 4 minutes.

Scrape the onions, garlic, and butter into your blender or food processor. Add everything else, and run until the onion and garlic disappear.

Pour it back into the saucepan and bring to a simmer. Let it cook for 20 minutes or so. Put it in a clean jar or snap-top container and store in the fridge.

Yield: 2½ cups (600 g), or 20 servings, each with 47 Calories; 3 g Fat; 1 g Protein; 7 g Carbohydrate; 1 g Dietary Fiber; 6 g Net Carbs.

Sauce Mornay

1 cup (235 ml) heavy cream

1 tablespoon (10 g) minced shallot

1 egg yolk

2 tablespoons (16 g) shredded Gruyère cheese

2 tablespoons (10 g) shredded Parmesan cheese

Dash of hot sauce

¼ teaspoon salt

This de-carbed version of a classic sauce is beyond luscious. Great on asparagus, broccoli, eggs, fish, chicken, shirataki, zoodles, fingers, you name it.

In a double boiler, over hot-but-not-boiling water, start the cream warming with the shallot in it.

When the cream is just below simmering—the surface will shimmer just a bit—whisk ¼ cup (60 ml) of it into the egg yolk. Then whisk the cream-and-yolk mixture back into the cream. Do not try to simply whisk the yolk into the main pot of cream or your sauce will fall apart instead of thickening.

Whisk in the two cheeses. Keep whisking as the sauce thickens, which will happen quickly.

Stir in the hot sauce and salt, and your sauce is done. Try to refrain from simply eating it all out of the pot.

Yield: 1¼ cups (295 ml), or 5 servings, each with 197 Calories; 20 g Fat; 3 g Protein; 2 g Carbohydrate; trace Dietary Fiber; 2 g Net Carbs.

Citrus Ham Glaze

¼ cup (60 g) Polaner sugar-free orange marmalade

2 tablespoons (40 g) sugar-free imitation honey (see Note)

1 tablespoon (15 ml) grapefruit-infused balsamic vinegar (see Note)

1 tablespoon (15 ml) lime juice

1 tablespoon (11 g) Dijon mustard

Pinch of ground cloves

As I put the finishing touches on this book, Easter left me with a half ham. ("Half a ham" sounds like leftovers. I bought a half ham.) It comes with a packet of sugary glaze that takes the carb count up to 4 grams per serving, which is high for meat. This will reduce the carb count, and it tastes better, too. It's also great on chicken or seafood.

Combine everything in a nonreactive saucepan and whisk over low heat until you have an even mixture. Use it just like any glaze.

Yield: 6 servings, each with 9 Calories; trace Fat; trace Protein; 3 g Carbohydrate; 2 g Dietary Fiber; 1 g Net Carbs.

RECIPE NOTE

- Sugar-free imitation honey, a honey-flavored syrup of maltitol or xylitol, depending on the brand, has become pretty widely available at local grocery stores, and I hear Walmart carries it. Like real honey, it keeps for just about forever. I like HoneyTree brand.

- If you're feeling creative, put ¼ of a ruby grapefruit, skin and all, in a nonreactive saucepan with 2 cups (470 ml) of balsamic vinegar. Bring to a low simmer, and let it cook until the vinegar is reduced by at least 25 percent. Now squeeze all the juice from the grapefruit quarter into the vinegar; let it cool, bottle, and use. It's lovely on salads.

- A third option is to buy good-quality balsamic and add a few drops of grapefruit essential oil; I get this at my health food store.

Horseradish Mustard Sauce

½ cup (120 g) sour cream

2½ tablespoons (26 g) horseradish mustard (I use Koops')

Salt and pepper, to taste

Want to liven up a steak with virtually no effort? This will do it! It's good on hamburgers, too, or as a dip for asparagus or artichokes.

Just stir the sour cream and horseradish mustard together and add a little salt and pepper to taste. Spoon this over a freshly grilled steak.

Yield: 4 servings, each with 70 Calories; 7 g Fat; 1 g Protein; 2 g Carbohydrate; trace Dietary Fiber; 2 g Net Carbs.

....

Creamy Sun-Dried Tomato and Pesto Sauce

½ cup (120 ml) heavy cream

2 tablespoons (30 g) pesto

2 tablespoons (20 g) oil-packed sun-dried tomatoes

I invented this for shirataki (page 87) or zoodles (page 124), but it would be aces on chicken, as well. And it's super quick and easy!

It can't get any easier: put everything in your food processor, and process until the tomatoes are pulverized. Done.

Yield: 4 servings, each with 148 Calories; 15 g Fat; 2 g Protein; 2 g Carbohydrate; trace Dietary Fiber; 2 g Net Carbs.

Sesame Sauce

½ cup (120 g) tahini
(sesame seed butter)

8 teaspoons (40 ml)
lemon juice

2 cloves of garlic

½ teaspoon cumin

¼ teaspoon cayenne

½ teaspoon dark sesame oil

½ cup (120 ml) water,
or as desired

Salt and pepper, to taste

2 tablespoons (7.5 g)
minced parsley

Delicious and unusual, this sauce is wonderful tossed with steamed broccoli, but try it with lamb or chicken, too.

Put the tahini, lemon juice, garlic, cumin, cayenne, and dark sesame oil in your food processor and process, scraping down the sides from time to time, until it's all well combined and the garlic is pulverized.

With the processor running, add the water 1 tablespoon (15 ml) at a time. Again, you may want to stop the processor and scrape down the sides once or twice. I use ¼ cup (60 ml) of water, but you can use more or less until you have the consistency you want. Mine was thick and creamy.

Season with salt and pepper to taste. Add the minced parsley and run the processor until it's just worked in. That's it!

Yield: 1 cup (240 g), or 4 servings, each with 190 Calories; 17 g Fat; 5 g Protein; 8 g Carbohydrate; 3 g Dietary Fiber; 5 g Net Carbs.

DESSERTS

I approach desserts with mixed feelings. While the ideal is to stop making sweets a regular part of your diet, for many people the knowledge that a dessert is fine from time to time is what allows them to embrace this dietary change.

From the perspective of preventing or treating insulin resistance, there are big differences among desserts. People assume the main problem is sugar, but that is not always the case. Many sweets contain more starch than sugar: cakes, cookies, doughnuts, pastries—pretty much anything made with flour—not to mention puddings, which are made with cornstarch or arrowroot. These desserts are far worse for you than, say, a scoop of ice cream (without cookie dough or brownie chunks or the like), or a few squares of dark chocolate. Look for no-sugar-added ice cream, ice pops, and fudge pops. (Skip the no-sugar-added ice cream sandwiches—they have flour in the cookies.)

Sugar-free candy has become ubiquitous, and I am happy to report that sugar-free Reese's peanut butter cups taste just like the originals and Russell Stover's sugar-free toffee squares are a dead ringer for Heath bars. However, a word of warning: virtually all of these commercially produced sugar-free sweets use maltitol because it behaves like sugar in cooking, giving all the textures and flavors sugar does. In fairly modest quantities, maltitol can give you gas. In larger quantities, it is a laxative. I can get away with one or two sugar-free mini peanut butter cups or toffee squares per day, but if I eat more I will regret it. So will you, especially if you have a job interview, a hot date, or plan on flying.

Much of ice cream is made up of milk and cream. Accordingly, the sugar-free versions will have a relatively modest quantity of maltitol. But candies like jelly beans, taffies, and hard candies are made almost entirely of sugar. This means that their sugar-free counterparts will consist almost entirely of maltitol. You might as well think of sugar-free jelly beans and gummies as particularly tasty laxative tablets. Eat more than two or three at your peril.

With this in mind, I offer you a few recipes that will replace sweets that are not only sugary but starchy as well. I think you'll be astonished at just how good they are. After all, flour has no flavor. But almond meal and vanilla whey protein taste good in their own right, and bring extra richness to the flavor of these treats.

Fudgy Chocolate Whatchamacallit

4 eggs, at room temperature

Pinch of cream of tartar

½ cup (120 g) Swerve or erythritol

¼ teaspoon vanilla liquid stevia

½ cup (112 g) butter, melted

1 teaspoon vanilla extract

3 tablespoons (18 g) almond meal

3 tablespoons (24 g) vanilla whey protein powder

6 tablespoons (36 g) cocoa powder

2 cups (470 ml) half-and-half, lukewarm

This is not quite a cake, not quite a brownie, but very definitely chocolate-y good!

Preheat the oven to 325°F (170°C, or gas mark 3). Grease an 8 × 8-inch (20 × 20 cm) baking pan or coat it with nonstick cooking spray.

Separate one egg at a time, letting the white flow into a custard cup, and dumping the yolk into a larger mixing bowl. Then dump the yolk-free whites into a deep, narrow bowl, and repeat, until all four whites are in one mixing bowl and the yolks in the other.

Add a small pinch of cream of tartar to the whites, and use an electric mixer to whip at highest speed until they're stiff. Set aside.

To the yolks in the other bowl add the Swerve and stevia. At medium speed, use your mixer to beat the yolks and sweeteners for 2 to 3 minutes, until light. There's no need to remove any of the white part (whereas even a tiny bit of yolk will mess up whipped egg whites).

Now add the melted butter a little at a time, beating the whole time. Beat in the vanilla extract, too.

A tablespoon (6 g) at a time, beat in the almond meal, vanilla whey protein, and then the cocoa powder. Scrape down the sides often, and keep beating until it's all well incorporated.

Little by little, start beating in the half-and-half. When all the half-and-half is in, turn off the mixer. The mixture will be thin and runny. Do not panic.

Add about one-third of the whipped egg whites to the batter, and, using a rubber scraper, fold them in gently. Repeat with the next third, then the last third.

Pour into the prepared baking pan, and bake for 50 minutes. Cool and chill before cutting. Serve with whipped cream!

Yield: 9 servings, each with 229 Calories; 20 g Fat; 10 g Protein; 6 g Carbohydrate; 1 g Dietary Fiber; 5 g Net Carbs.

Chocolate Chip Cookies

1 cup (95 g) almond meal

1 cup (128 g) vanilla whey protein powder

1 teaspoon baking soda

1 teaspoon salt

1 cup (225 g) butter, at room temperature

1 cup (240 g) erythritol

2 teaspoons molasses

½ teaspoon English toffee liquid stevia

2 eggs

1 cup (110 g) chopped pecans

12 ounces (340 g) no-sugar-added chocolate chips

I often introduce myself by saying, "If you want to know how to make a sugar-free, flourless chocolate chip cookie that tastes like a chocolate chip cookie, I'm your girl."

Preheat the oven to 375°F (190°C, or gas mark 5). Line 2 cookie sheets with baking parchment.

In a medium-size mixing bowl, stir together the almond meal, vanilla whey protein, baking soda, and salt until everything is evenly distributed.

In a larger mixing bowl, using an electric mixer, beat the butter with the erythritol, molasses, and liquid stevia until light and fluffy.

Beat in the eggs one at a time, letting the first one get incorporated before adding the second. Now beat in the almond meal/vanilla whey mixture, in three additions. When all the dry ingredients are worked in, fold in the pecans and chocolate chips.

Scoop by the tablespoon (15 g) onto the prepared cookie sheets. Bake for 10 to 12 minutes, or until golden. Transfer to wire racks to cool.

Yield: 54 cookies, each with 76 Calories; 6 g Fat; 4 g Protein; 1 g Carbohydrate; trace Dietary Fiber; 1 g Net Carbs.

RECIPE NOTE

There are a few brands of sugar-free chocolate chips out there. I like Lily's, which are sweetened with stevia and erythritol, but Hershey's makes a maltitol-sweetened version (see warnings about maltitol on page 170). You can also chop sugar-free semisweet chocolate into chip-size bits in your food processor.

Peanut-Coco-Chocolate-Chip Cookies

1⅓ cups (126 g) almond meal

1⅓ cups (170 g) vanilla whey protein powder

1⅓ cups (115 g) shredded coconut meat

2 teaspoons baking soda

2 teaspoons salt

1 cup (225 g) butter, at room temperature

1 cup (260 g) natural peanut butter

1 cup (25 g) Splenda

⅔ cup (160 g) erythritol

4 teaspoons (27 g) molasses

1 tablespoon (15 ml) vanilla extract

4 eggs

2 cups (350 g) no-sugar-added chocolate chips

I love peanuts and chocolate together. Doesn't everyone?

Preheat the oven to 375°F (190°C, or gas mark 5). Spray cookie sheets with nonstick cooking spray, or line with baking parchment or other nonstick pan liners.

In a large bowl, combine the almond meal, vanilla whey protein, coconut, baking soda, and salt and stir together until everything is well distributed.

In a separate bowl, using an electric mixer, beat together the butter and peanut butter thoroughly. Now add the Splenda, erythritol, and molasses, and beat until fluffy.

Add the vanilla, then the eggs, one at a time, beating well after each addition.

When the eggs are thoroughly incorporated, add the dry ingredients, about one-third of the mixture at a time, beating well after each addition. Don't forget to scrape down the sides of the bowl now and then!

Finally, stir in the chocolate chips.

Scoop onto the prepared cookie sheets. I use a cookie scoop—like an ice cream scoop, only smaller; each cookie uses 2 tablespoons (30 g) of dough. Keep in mind that they don't spread a lot; mine came out in nice rounded, ball shapes, just as they came out of the cookie scoop. Of course, you can flatten them if you want.

Bake for 12 minutes, or until golden, keeping in mind that if you are making yours smaller than my 2-tablespoon (30 g) scoops, they'll take a bit less time. Cool on a wire rack and store in a snap-top container.

Yield: 56 cookies, each with 150 Calories; 10 g Fat; 7 g Protein; 8 g Carbohydrate; 5 g Dietary Fiber; 3 g Net Carbs.

German Chocolate Chip Cookies

1 cup (85 g) shredded coconut meat

⅔ cup (60 g) almond meal

⅔ cup (85 g) vanilla whey protein powder

1 tablespoon (6 g) cocoa powder

1 teaspoon baking soda

½ teaspoon baking powder

½ teaspoon salt

½ cup (112 g) butter, at room temperature

½ cup (112 g) coconut oil, at room temperature

¾ cup (180 g) erythritol

½ teaspoon vanilla liquid stevia

2 eggs

2 cups (350 g) no-sugar-added chocolate chips

½ cup (55 g) chopped pecans

Remember that starches have no flavor, but our ingredients do! That's what makes these cookies so mind-blowingly great.

Preheat the oven to 350°F (180°C, or gas mark 4). Line 2 cookie sheets with baking parchment.

Combine the coconut, almond meal, vanilla whey protein, cocoa powder, baking soda, baking powder, and salt in a bowl, stirring well, so everything is evenly distributed.

In another bowl, using an electric mixer, beat together the butter and coconut oil. Now beat in the erythritol in three additions. Beat until well blended and fluffy. Add the stevia, and beat in in.

Beat in the eggs, one at a time, incorporating the first well before adding the second.

When both eggs are beaten in, beat in the dry ingredients in three or four additions.

Turn the mixer to low speed, and beat in the chocolate chips and pecans.

I scooped the dough with a cookie scoop; the 40 count is based on 2-tablespoon (30 g) cookies. Scoop the dough onto cookie sheets, leaving room for spreading.

Bake for 12 minutes, but check at 10; oven thermometers aren't always accurate. Transfer to a wire rack to cool, and store in a tightly lidded container.

Yield: 40 cookies, each with 152 Calories; 12 g Fat; 5 g Protein; 8 g Carbohydrate; 6 g Dietary Fiber; 2 g Net Carbs.

APPENDIX

GLYCEMIC LOADS
(Expressed as percentage of the glycemic load of a 1-oz [28 g] slice of white bread)

Food item	Description	Glycemic index	Available carbohydrate (percent)	Typical American serving	Glycemic load
Baked goods					
Oatmeal cookie	1 medium	77	68	1 oz (28 g)	102
Apple muffin, sugarless	2½-inch (6.4 cm) diameter	69	32	2½ oz (70 g)	107
Cookie: average, all types	1 medium	84	64	1 oz (28 g)	114
Croissant	1 medium	96	46	1½ oz (42 g)	127
Crumpet	1 medium	69	38	2 oz (56 g)	148
Bran muffin	2½-inch (6.4 cm) diameter	85	42	2 oz (56 g)	149
Pastry	1 serving (3 × 3 × 1-inch [7.5 × 7.5 × 2.5 cm])	84	46	2 oz (56 g)	149
Chocolate cake	1 slice (4 × 4 × 1-inch [10 × 10 × 2.5 cm])	54	47	3 oz (84 g)	154
Vanilla wafers	4 wafers	110	72	1 oz (28 g)	159
Graham cracker	1 rectangle	106	72	1 oz (28 g)	159
Blueberry muffin	2½-inch (6.4 cm) diameter	84	51	2 oz (56 g)	169
Pita bread	1 medium	82	57	2 oz (56 g)	189
Carrot cake	1 square (3 × 3 × 1½-inch [7.5 × 7.5 × 3.8 cm])	88	56	2 oz (56 g)	199
Carrot muffin	2½-inch (6.4 cm) diameter	88	56	2 oz (56 g)	199
Waffle	7-inch (18 cm) diameter	109	37	2½ oz (70 g)	203
Doughnut	1 medium	108	49	2 oz (56 g)	205
Cupcake	2½-inch (6.4 cm) diameter	104	68	1½ oz (42 g)	213
Angel food cake	1 slice (4 × 4 × 1-inch [10 × 10 × 2.5 cm])	95	58	2 oz (56 g)	216
English muffin	1 medium	109	47	2 oz (56 g)	224

(continued)

Food item	Description	Glycemic index	Available carbohydrate (percent)	Typical American serving	Glycemic load
Pound cake	1 slice (4 × 4 × 1-inch [10 × 10 × 2.5 cm])	77	53	3 oz (84 g)	241
Corn muffin	2½-inch (6.4 cm) diameter	146	51	2 oz (56 g)	299
Pancake	5-inch (12.5 cm) diameter	96	73	2½ oz (70 g)	346
Alcoholic beverages					
Spirits	1½ oz (45 ml)	< 15		1½ oz (45 ml)	< 15
Red wine	6-oz (180 ml) glass	< 15		6 oz (180 ml)	< 15
White wine	6-oz (180 ml) glass	< 15		6 oz (180 ml)	< 15
Beer	12-oz (360 ml) can/bottle	< 15		12 oz (360 ml)	70
Nonalcoholic beverages					
Tomato juice	6-oz (180 ml) glass	54	4	6 oz (180 ml)	27
V8 juice	6-oz (180 ml) glass	61	4	6 oz (180 ml)	27
Carrot juice	6-oz (180 ml) glass	61	12	6 oz (180 ml)	68
Grapefruit juice, unsweetened	6-oz (180 ml) glass	69	9	6 oz (180 ml)	75
Apple juice, unsweetened	6-oz (180 ml) glass	57	12	6 oz (180 ml)	82
Chocolate milk	8-oz (235 ml) glass	49	10	8 oz (235 ml)	82
Orange juice	6-oz (180 ml) glass	71	10	6 oz (180 ml)	89
Prune juice	6-oz (180 ml) glass	61	14	6 oz (180 ml)	102
Cranberry juice	6-oz (180 ml) glass	80	12	6 oz (180 ml)	109
Pineapple juice, unsweetened	6-oz (180 ml) glass	66	14	6 oz (180 ml)	109
Raspberry smoothie	8-oz (235 ml) glass	48	16	8 oz (235 ml)	127
Lemonade	8-oz (235 ml) glass	77	11	8 oz (235 ml)	136
Ensure	8-oz (235 ml) glass	71	17	8 oz (235 ml)	182
Coca-Cola	12-oz (360 ml) can	90	10	12 oz (360 ml)	218
Gatorade	20-oz (600 ml) bottle	111	6	20 oz (600 ml)	273
Orange soda	12-oz (355 ml) glass	97	14	12 oz (355 ml)	314
Breads and rolls					
Tortilla (wheat)	1 medium	43	52	1⅜ oz (40 g)	64
Pizza crust	1 slice	43	22	3½ oz (98 g)	70

(continued)

Food item	Description	Glycemic index	Available carbohydrate (percent)	Typical American serving	Glycemic load
Tortilla (corn)	1 medium	74	48	1¼ oz (35 g)	87
White bread	½-inch (1.3 cm) slice	100	47	1 oz (28 g)	107
Whole-meal rye bread	⅜-inch (1 cm) slice	97	40	2 oz (56 g)	114
Sourdough bread	⅜-inch (1 cm) slice	77	47	1½ oz (42 g)	114
Oat bran bread	⅜-inch (1 cm) slice	68	60	1½ oz (42 g)	128
Whole-wheat bread	½-inch (1.3 cm) slice	101	43	1½ oz (42 g)	129
Rye bread	⅜-inch (1 cm) slice	97	47	1½ oz (42 g)	142
Banana bread, sugarless	1 slice (4 × 4 × 1-inch [10 × 10 × 2.5 cm])	79	48	3 oz (84 g)	170
80% whole-kernel oat bread	⅜-inch (1 cm) slice	93	63	1½ oz (42 g)	170
Buckwheat bread	⅜-inch (1 cm) slice	95	63	1½ oz (42 g)	183
80% whole-kernel barley bread	⅜-inch (1 cm) slice	95	67	1½ oz (42 g)	185
Pita bread	8-inch (20 cm) diameter	82	57	2 oz (56 g)	189
Hamburger bun	Top and bottom, 5-inch (12.5 cm) diameter	87	50	2½ oz (70 g)	213
80% whole-kernel wheat bread	⅜-inch (1 cm) slice	74	67	2¼ oz (63 g)	213
French bread	½-inch (1.3 cm) slice	136	50	2 oz (56 g)	284
Bagel	1 medium	103	50	3⅓ oz (99 g)	340
Breakfast cereals					
All-Bran	½ cup (28 g)	54	77	1 oz (28 g)	85
Muesli	1 cup (28 g)	69	53	1 oz (28 g)	95
Oatmeal (from rolled oats)	1 cup (227 g)	80	10	8 oz (227 g)	123
Special K	1 cup (28 g)	98	70	1 oz (28 g)	133
Cheerios	1 cup (28 g)	106	40	1 oz (28 g)	142
Shredded Wheat	1 cup (28 g)	107	67	1 oz (28 g)	142
Grape-Nuts	1 cup (116 g)	102	70	4 oz (116 g)	142
Granola	1 cup (28 g)	90	87	1 oz (28 g)	142

(continued)

Food item	Description	Glycemic index	Available carbohydrate (percent)	Typical American serving	Glycemic load
Puffed wheat	1 cup (28 g)	105	70	1 oz (28 g)	151
Kashi	1 cup (28 g)	93	80	1 oz (28 g)	151
Instant oatmeal	1 cup (227 g)	94	10	8 oz (227 g)	154
Cream of Wheat, cooked	1 cup (227 g)	94	10	8 oz (227 g)	154
Total	1 cup (28 g)	109	73	1 oz (28 g)	161
Froot Loops	1 cup (28 g)	98	87	1 oz (28 g)	170
Corn Flakes	1 cup (28 g)	116	77	1 oz (28 g)	199
Rice Krispies	1 cup (28 g)	117	87	1 oz (28 g)	208
Rice Chex	1 cup (28 g)	127	87	1 oz (28 g)	218
Raisin Bran	1 cup (56 g)	87	63	2 oz (56 g)	227
Candy					
Sugar-free milk chocolate	2 squares (1 × 1 × ¼-inch [2.5 × 2.5 × 0.6 cm])			1 oz (28 g)	17
Lifesaver	1 piece	100	100	¹⁄₁₀ oz (2.8 g)	20
Dark chocolate	2 squares (1 × 1 × ¼-inch [2.5 × 2.5 × 0.6 cm])			1 oz (28 g)	44
Peanut M&Ms	1 snack-size package	47	57	¾ oz (21 g)	43
Licorice	1 twist	111	70	⅓ oz (9 g)	45
White chocolate	2 squares (1 × 1 × ¼-inch [2.5 × 2.5 × 0.6 cm])	63	44	⅔ oz (18 g)	49
Milk chocolate	2 squares (1 × 1 × ¼-inch [2.5 × 2.5 × 0.6 cm])	61	44	1 oz (28 g)	68
Jelly beans	6 beans	112	93	½ oz (14 g)	104
Granola bar, apple, cranberry	1 bar	82	77	1 oz (28 g)	131
Snickers bar	1 regular size bar	97	57	2 oz (56 g)	218
Chips and crackers					
Potato chips	Small bag	77	42	1 oz (28 g)	62
Corn chips	1 package	90	52	1 oz (28 g)	97
Popcorn	4 cups (28 g)	103	55	1 oz (28 g)	114
Rye crisps	1 rectangle	91	64	1 oz (28 g)	125
Wheat Thins	4 small	96	68	1 oz (28 g)	136

(continued)

Food item	Description	Glycemic index	Available carbohydrate (percent)	Typical American serving	Glycemic load
Soda cracker	2 regular size	106	68	1 oz (28 g)	136
Pretzels	Small bag	119	67	1 oz (28 g)	151
Rice cakes	3 regular size	117	84	1 oz (28 g)	190
Dairy products					
Cheese	1 slice (2 × 2 × 1-inch [5 × 5 × 2.5 cm])	< 15	0	2 oz (56 g)	< 15
Butter	1 tablespoon (14 g)	< 15	0	½ oz (14 g)	< 15
Margarine	Typical serving	< 15	0	¼ oz (7 g)	< 15
Sour cream	Typical serving	< 15	0	2 oz (56 g)	< 15
Yogurt, full fat (unsweetened)	½ cup (112 g)	51	5	4 oz (112 g)	17
Milk (whole)	8-oz (235 ml) glass	49	5	8 oz (235 ml)	37
Milk (skim)	8-oz (235 ml) glass	50	5	8 oz (235 ml)	41
Yogurt, low fat (sweetened)	½ cup (112 g)	47	16	4 oz (112 g)	57
Soymilk	8-oz (235 ml) glass	60	7	8 oz (235 ml)	62
Vanilla ice cream (high fat)	½ cup (112 g)	54	18	4 oz (112 g)	68
Milk (low-fat chocolate)	8-oz (235 ml) glass	49	10	8 oz (235 ml)	82
Custard	½ cup (130 g)	61	17	4½ oz (130 g)	89
Chocolate pudding	½ cup (130 g)	67	16	4½ oz (130 g)	89
Chocolate ice cream (high fat)	½ cup (130 g)	53	18	4½ oz (130 g)	91
Vanilla ice cream (low fat)	½ cup (112 g)	58	36	4 oz (112 g)	159
Frozen tofu	½ cup (112 g)	164	30	4 oz (112 g)	379
Fruit					
Strawberries	1 cup (154 g)	57	3	5½ oz (154 g)	13
Apricot	1 medium	82	8	2 oz (56 g)	24
Grapefruit	1 half	36	9	4½ oz (130 g)	32
Plum	1 medium	55	10	3 oz (84 g)	36
Nectarine	1 medium	61	8	4 oz (112 g)	38

(continued)

Food item	Description	Glycemic index	Available carbohydrate (percent)	Typical American serving	Glycemic load
Cherries, dark	8 cherries	90	12	2 oz (56 g)	43
Kiwi	1 medium	75	10	3 oz (84 g)	43
Peach, canned in natural juice	½ cup (112 g)	58	10	4 oz (112 g)	45
Peach, fresh	1 medium	60	9	4 oz (112 g)	47
Grapes	½ cup (70 g)	66	15	2½ oz (70 g)	47
Pineapple	1 slice (¾ × 3½-inches [2 × 9 cm])	59	11	3 oz (84 g)	50
Watermelon	1 cup (154 g) cubed	103	5	5½ oz (154 g)	52
Cantaloupe	1 cup (154 g) cubed	93	5	5½ oz (154 g)	52
Pear	1 medium	54	9	6 oz (168 g)	57
Mango	½ cup (84 g)	73	14	3 oz (84 g)	57
Orange	1 medium	60	9	6 oz (168 g)	71
Apricot, dried	2 oz (56 g)	43	45	2 oz (56 g)	76
Apple	1 medium	52	13	5½ oz (154 g)	78
Banana	1 medium	74	17	3¼ oz (91 g)	85
Prunes, pitted, dried	2 oz (56 g)	41	55	2 oz (56 g)	95
Apple, dried	2 oz (56 g)	41	60	2 oz (56 g)	104
Peach, canned in heavy syrup	½ cup (112 g)	92	16	4 oz (112 g)	112
Raisins	2 tablespoons (28 g)	91	73	1 oz (28 g)	133
Figs	3 medium	87	43	2 oz (56 g)	151
Dates	5 medium	147	67	1½ oz (42 g)	298
Meat					
Beef	10-oz (280 g) steak	< 15		10 oz (280 g)	< 15
Pork	Two 5-oz (140 g) chops	< 15		10 oz (280 g)	< 15
Chicken	1 breast	< 15		10 oz (280 g)	< 15
Fish	8-oz (227 g) fillet	< 15		8 oz (227 g)	< 15
Lamb	Three 4-oz (112 g) chops	< 15		12 oz (340 g)	< 15
Mixed meals					
Deluxe burger, no bun	1 medium			3¼ oz (91 g)	< 15

(continued)

Food item	Description	Glycemic index	Available carbohydrate (percent)	Typical American serving	Glycemic load
Pizza, minus outer rim of crust	1 slice	51	12	3 oz (84 g)	45
Wheat tortilla, bean filled	1 tube	40	18	4 oz (112 g)	50
Chicken nuggets	4 oz (112 g)	66	16	4 oz (112 g)	70
Deluxe burger, no top bun	1 medium	47	8	4¼ oz (119 g)	80
Cannelloni, spinach & ricotta	2 tubes	21	18	12 oz (340 g)	88
Pizza, crust intact	1 slice	51	24	4 oz (112 g)	90
Chili con carne	1 cup (227 g)	49	12	8 oz (227 g)	91
Veggie burger	1 medium	84	24	3½ oz (98 g)	140
Deluxe hamburger	1 medium	94	16	5¾ oz (160 g)	170
Fillet-O-Fish	1 medium	94	30	4½ oz (126 g)	200
Chicken korma and rice	10 oz (280 g)	63	16	10 oz (280 g)	210
McChicken	1 medium	94	22	6½ oz (182 g)	260
Nuts					
Peanuts	¼ cup (35 g)	21	8	1¼ oz (35 g)	< 15
Walnuts	¼ cup (35 g)	20	8	1¼ oz (35 g)	< 15
Almonds	¼ cup (35 g)	20	8	1¼ oz (35 g)	< 15
Cashews	¼ cup (35 g)	31	26	1¼ oz (35 g)	21
Pasta					
Asian bean noodles	1 cup (140 g)	47	25	5 oz (140 g)	118
Spaghetti, whole grain	1 cup (140 g)	53	23	5 oz (140 g)	126
Vermicelli	1 cup (140 g)	50	24	5 oz (140 g)	126
Spaghetti (boiled 5 minutes)	1 cup (140 g)	54	27	5 oz (140 g)	142
Fettuccine	1 cup (140 g)	57	23	5 oz (140 g)	142

(continued)

Food item	Description	Glycemic index	Available carbohydrate (percent)	Typical American serving	Glycemic load
Noodles (instant, boiled 2 minutes)	1 cup (140 g)	67	22	5 oz (140 g)	150
Capellini	1 cup (140 g)	64	25	5 oz (140 g)	158
Spaghetti (boiled 10 to 15 minutes)	1 cup (140 g)	64	27	5 oz (140 g)	166
Linguine	1 cup (140 g)	74	25	5 oz (140 g)	181
Macaroni	1 cup (140 g)	67	28	5 oz (140 g)	181
Rice noodles	1 cup (140 g)	87	22	5 oz (140 g)	181
Spaghetti (boiled 20 minutes)	1 cup (140 g)	87	24	5 oz (140 g)	213
Macaroni and cheese (boxed)	1 cup (140 g)	92	28	5 oz (140 g)	252
Gnocchi	1 cup (140 g)	97	27	5 oz (140 g)	260
Soups					
Tomato	1 cup (227 g)	54	7	8 oz (227 g)	55
Minestrone	1 cup (227 g)	56	7	8 oz (227 g)	64
Lentil	1 cup (227 g)	63	8	8 oz (227 g)	82
Split pea	1 cup (227 g)	86	11	8 oz (227 g)	145
Black bean	1 cup (227 g)	92	11	8 oz (227 g)	154
Sweeteners					
Artificial sweeteners	1 teaspoon (5 g)	< 15		⅙ oz (5 g)	< 15
Honey	1 teaspoon (5 g)	78	72	⅙ oz (5 g)	16
Table sugar	1 round teaspoon (5 g)	97	100	⅙ oz (5 g)	28
Syrup	¼ cup (56 g)	97		2 oz (56 g)	364
Vegetables					
Lettuce	1 cup (70 g)	< 15		2½ oz (70 g)	< 15
Spinach	1 cup (70 g)	< 15		2½ oz (70 g)	< 15
Cucumber	1 cup (168 g)	< 15		6 oz (168 g)	< 15
Mushrooms	½ cup (56 g)	< 15		2 oz (56 g)	< 15
Asparagus	4 spears	< 15		3 oz (84 g)	< 15
Peppers	½ medium	< 15		2 oz (56 g)	< 15
Broccoli	½ cup (42 g)	< 15		1½ oz (42 g)	< 15

(continued)

Food item	Description	Glycemic index	Available carbohydrate (percent)	Typical American serving	Glycemic load
Carrot (raw)	1 medium (7½ inch [19 cm])	23	10	3 oz (84 g)	11
Tomato	1 medium	< 15		5 oz (140 g)	< 15
Peas	¼ cup (42 g)	68	9	1½ oz (42 g)	16
Chickpeas, boiled	½ cup (84 g)	14	20	3 oz (84 g)	17
Carrot, boiled	⅔ cup (84 g)	70	6	3 oz (84 g)	21
Fava beans	½ cup (84 g)	90	6	3 oz (84 g)	32
Lentils	½ cup (98 g)	42	11	3½ oz (98 g)	33
Butter beans	½ cup (84 g)	44	13	3 oz (84 g)	34
Cannellini beans	½ cup (84 g)	44	14	3 oz (84 g)	34
Kidney beans	½ cup (84 g)	39	17	3 oz (84 g)	40
Navy beans	½ cup (84 g)	69	10	3 oz (84 g)	40
Beets	½ cup (112 g)	80	63	4 oz (112 g)	50
Parsnips	½ cup (84 g)	74	10	3 oz (84 g)	50
Lima beans	½ cup (84 g)	46	12	3 oz (84 g)	57
Refried pinto beans	½ cup (84 g)	55	17	3 oz (84 g)	57
Black-eyed beans	½ cup (84 g)	59	20	3 oz (84 g)	74
Yam	½ cup (140 g)	53	24	5 oz (140 g)	123
Quinoa	1 cup (182 g)	76	17	6½ oz (182 g)	160
Potato (instant, mashed)	¾ cup (140 g)	122	13	5 oz (140 g)	161
Sweet potato	½ cup (140 g)	87	19	5 oz (140 g)	161
Corn on the cob	1 ear	78	21	5⅓ oz (150 g)	171
Couscous	½ cup (112 g)	93	23	4 oz (112 g)	174
Rice cakes	1 medium	110	84	1 oz (28 g)	193
French fries (McDonald's)	1 large serving	107	19	5.9 oz (168 g)	219
Brown and wild rice mix	1 cup (182 g)	64	26	6½ oz (182 g)	221
Brown rice	1 cup (182 g)	79	22	6½ oz (182 g)	222
Baked potato	1 medium	121	20	5 oz (140 g)	246
Basmati rice	1 cup (182 g)	83	25	6½ oz (182 g)	271

(continued)

Food item	Description	Glycemic index	Available carbohydrate (percent)	Typical American serving	Glycemic load
White rice	1 cup (182 g)	91	24	6½ oz (182 g)	283
Sticky white rice	1 cup (182 g)	124	19	6½ oz (182 g)	295
Miscellaneous					
Eggs	Typical serving	< 15		1½ oz (42 g)	< 15
Salad dressing	Typical serving	< 15		2 oz (56 g)	< 15
Agave	1 teaspoon (7 g)	< 15		¼ oz (7 g)	< 15
Cane sugar	1 level teaspoon (3.5 g)	94	100	⅛ oz (3.5 g)	28

Source: Rob Thompson, M.D. The glycemic loads in this book are expressed as percentages of the blood-glucose-raising effect of a single ¼-inch (6 mm) thick slice of white bread and reflect typical American servings, which sometimes differ from international listings. See page 43 for more information. Note: Per serving gram amounts may vary depending on source and food preparation methods.

ACKNOWLEDGMENTS

I would like to thank Laura Smith and Jill Alexander of Fair Winds Press for their editorial assistance in writing this book, and my agent, Roger Williams, for handling the contract details. I also owe a debt of gratitude to my now retired, former agent, Elizabeth Frost-Knappman, who first took an interest in my work. My old friend Robert E. (Gene) McIntosh, one of Seattle's leading fertility specialists, kept me on the right track in my discussion of polycystic ovary syndrome. If it weren't for my office staff, Shannon Brown and Caroline Brown, the best in town, I wouldn't have the time to write. Most of all, I owe thanks to my wife Kathy for her patience and support. *—Rob Thompson*

As always, thanks to my recipe testers. You guys are such a huge help! To Rob Thompson, for once again including me in his work and for being a thoroughly good guy. To Jill Alexander, for being patient with my periodic flakiness. And, forever, to my husband, Eric Schmitz, who supports my work in every way imaginable. I'd make a lot more grocery store runs and destroy a lot more computers without him. *—Dana Carpender*

ABOUT THE AUTHORS

Rob Thompson, M.D., is a board-certified internist and cardiologist who has been in full-time practice in Seattle for forty years. As a preventive cardiologist, he specializes in treating diseases that cause heart disease, including cholesterol imbalances, diabetes, and obesity. He is the author of several scientific articles on the treatment of heart disease. Other books written by him include *The New Low-Carb Way of Life*, *The Glycemic Load Diet*, *The Glycemic Load Diabetes Solution*, and *The Sugar Blockers Diet*.

In retrospect, **Dana Carpender**'s career seems inevitable: she has been cooking since she had to stand on a stepstool to reach the stove. She was also a dangerously sugar-addicted child, eventually stealing from her parents to support her habit, and was in Weight Watchers by age eleven. At nineteen, Dana read her first book on nutrition and recognized herself in a list of symptoms of reactive hypoglycemia. She ditched sugar and white flour, and was dazzled by the near-instantaneous improvement in her physical and mental health. A lifetime nutrition buff was born.

Unfortunately, in the late 1980s and early '90s, Dana got sucked into the low-fat/high-carb mania and whole-grain-and-beaned her way up to a size 20, with nasty energy swings, constant hunger, and borderline high blood pressure. In 1995, she read a nutrition book from the 1950s that stated that obesity had nothing to do with how much one ate, but was rather a carbohydrate intolerance disease. She thought, "What the heck, might as well give it a try." Three days later, her clothes were loose, her hunger was gone, and her energy level was through the roof. She never looked back, and has now been low-carb for nineteen years and counting—a third of her life.

Realizing that this change was permanent, and being a cook at heart, Dana set about creating as varied and satisfying a cuisine as she could with a minimal carb load. By 1997, she was writing about it, and now has more than 2,500 recipes published and more than a million books sold. Dana lives in Bloomington, Indiana, with her husband, three dogs, and a cat, all of whom are well and healthily fed.

INDEX